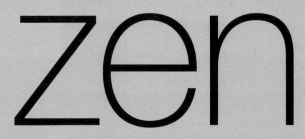

zen

and the art of

well-being

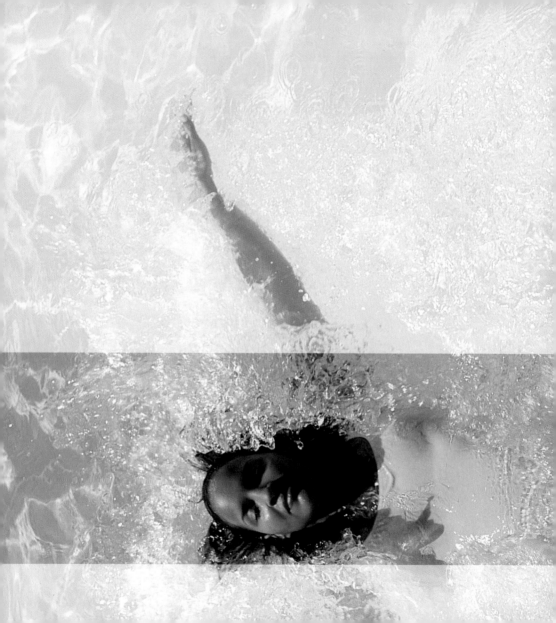

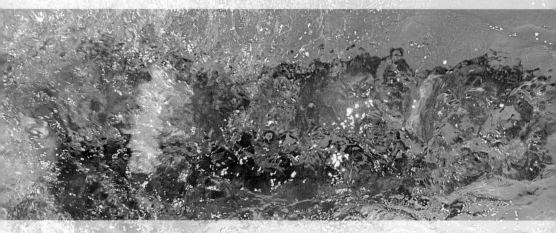

zen

and the art of
well-being

eric chaline

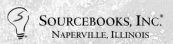

SOURCEBOOKS, INC.®
NAPERVILLE, ILLINOIS

contents

what is

"well-being"?

A decade ago, a book about well-being might have taken as its theme a number of different topics. If the author were a specialist in health and fitness, for example, he or she might focus on the physical aspects of well-being; alternatively, a psychologist or psychotherapist might concentrate on mental issues. Today, a book claiming to deal with well-being must embrace matters of both the mind and the body, as the two are now understood to be the inextricably connected parts of a single whole. This approach, known as "holism," has been popularized by "alternative therapies" that are often based on traditional Asian models of human health and fitness, such as India's Ayurveda (science of life) and traditional Chinese medicine.

When I was planning this book, I discussed the contents with a friend who is also my occasional editor. During one conversation, she remarked casually, "Oh, so you're writing a self-help book." I was shocked by the realization of this. Rather than writing a "how-to" book based on my experiences as a health and fitness consultant, with the "added value" of the inclusion of Zen Buddhist philosophy, the word "well-being" took it to a deeper level. It was clear I would have to draw on my own experiences and feelings about what "well-being" actually means to write a book that would be of any benefit to my readers.

I was reluctant to write a "self-help" book, but not because I have deep reservations about the whole genre. Being a member of the human race is qualification enough for anyone to write about his or her own direct experiences of life. But what often happens with "self-help" books—even those by the best-intentioned authors—is that they quickly turn into "tell-you-what-to-do" books. With depressing regularity, people who set themselves up as exemplars of one kind or another are proved to be fallible human beings: moral guardians, who are morally bankrupt or hypocritically mired in the "vices" they themselves condemn; health and fitness gurus who abuse their bodies in various ways.

Another school of "self-help" particularly prevalent in the United States is preached by the feel-good, self-empowerment gurus. They never tire of telling their readers that they can do anything—lose weight, quit smoking, fall in love, make friends, or earn a million dollars—if they only have a sufficiently positive mental attitude. This group is

the pitfalls of the self-help expert

probably even more dangerous than the "do-as-I-say" brigade, as they instill a sense of personal failure and guilt into readers who are not able to live up to their exacting combination of iron self-control and dynamic careerism.

There is yet a third class of self-help books. The authors of these books put forward truly original thinkers from the past or present—in other words, geniuses. Perhaps a genius can give good advice to other geniuses, but would you ask a Mozart or an Einstein to tell you how to improve your fitness or what to do when you get depressed?

I hope this book does not fall into any of these three classes of self-help book.

the Buddha

Gautama Siddharta, the historical Buddha, was, I believe, a uniquely gifted individual, but he was not a genius in the mold of Einstein or Mozart. When you strip away the myths that surround the historical figure, you find that Siddharta was a privileged and well-educated man, who, when confronted by the fundamental question of existence, was not satisfied with the answers that he had been taught.

The story of the Buddha's enlightenment is not one of a discovery born of precocious genius, but of hard slogging years of trial and error. The Buddha's quest was for much more than well-being. He sought enlightenment—that is, the complete understanding of the nature of reality. He first went to study with the leading scholars of the day, but having exhausted their wisdom, he concluded that the intellect alone would not give him the answers he sought. He then turned to the other path of spiritual inquiry that was open to men of his day: the physical yogas of the sadhu, or holy men. He retired to the forest, and his experiments with asceticism were so extreme that he almost died. But after seven years, so the legend goes, he abandoned asceticism, realizing that it would never lead him to enlightenment. He broke his fast and left the isolation of the forest, much to the disgust of his followers who had admired him for his erstwhile devotion.

His goal still eluding him, the Buddha sat down to meditate under a bodhi tree, determined to become enlightened or to die in the attempt. As the sun rose, after three days and nights of meditation, he became the Buddha, the enlightened one, and began his earthly ministry. Unlike many other prophets or messiahs, he did not issue commandments, write laws on stone tablets, or cast down the idols of rival gods. In his first sermon, he explained the Four Noble Truths, that give each of us an explanation of our unhappiness.

the four noble

truths

Life is suffering

Suffering is caused by selfish craving

Selfish craving can be overcome

If you follow the Eight-Fold Path

the eight-fold path

Is a practical method to attain enlightenment and the end of human suffering.

right thought

   right action

      right effort

         right speech

            right livelihood

               right attention

                  right concentration

                     right understanding

following the lead

There is much in the Buddha's life that exemplifies what *not* to do to gain enlightenment. In this, I feel confident that I can follow his lead, because there are many things in my own life that I can hold up as perfect examples of what not to do to attain or preserve well-being. Readers will not find any hard-and-fast prescriptions on how to attain well-being in the pages that follow, but they will find a wealth of practical information and first-hand experience of techniques that will help them make informed choices.

For the purposes of this book, I have divided well-being into three interrelated levels: physical, biochemical, and mental. The physical level includes the functions of the basic structural elements of the body, including the skeleton, musculature, and joints; the bio-chemical level includes all the invisible processes, such as respiration, digestion, and energy production; and the mental level comprises all the processes involving conscious thought, emotion, and belief.

The scientific understanding of the physical and biochemical levels is well advanced, and we now know how to promote well-being through diet and exercise. When it comes to the mental level, however, opinions are sharply divided. I will treat the mental level only in as far as it impacts the physical and biochemical levels, as it does so clearly in diet and stress. The effects of personal relationships, sexuality, work, and religious beliefs on well-being are determined by time, place, background, and culture, making it impossible to reach any practical conclusions or give advice.

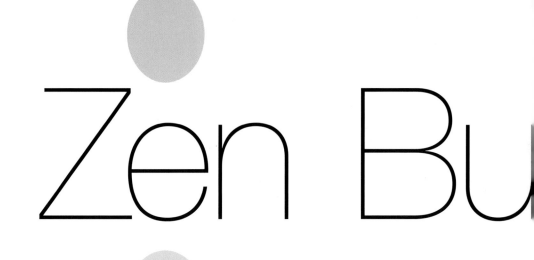

Zen Bu

ddhism

Zen Buddhism is devoted to the spiritual well-being of humanity, but in its concentration on the mental aspects of well-being; it does not overlook the physical and biochemical levels. Zen is an East-Asian philosophy, and it reflects the cultures in which it developed. Originating in India in the teaching of dhyana (meditation), or Ch'an in Chinese, Zen was brought to China by the monk Bodhidharma (470–534), a semi-legendary figure, who is said to have reached South China in 517 after a three-year journey. During its development in China, Ch'an was influenced by the native doctrines of the Tao—the Way—and of the interplay of the elemental forces of yin and yang, on which holistic theories of traditional Chinese medicine are based.

Ch'an came to Japan as Zen as early as the seventh century, but it did not develop a major following until the twelfth century when the monk Eisai (1141–1215) founded the Rinzai Zen sect and built the first Zen temple. The sect owed its success to its appeal to the samurai military elite, which had taken over the government of the country from the imperial aristocracy in 1185. Zen was patronized by the military ruler of Japan, the shogun Minamoto Yoriie. He appointed Eisai as Abbot of Kenninji in Kyoto in 1204, creating the first Zen monastery. The second major Japanese Zen sect, the Soto, was founded in 1243 by Dogen (1200–1253).

the fighting arts

It might seem strange to the modern reader that a Buddhist sect preaching absolute detachment from the world through meditation might find favor with a feudal military aristocracy. But the choice for the samurai caste was a purely pragmatic one. The spiritual discipline and austerity of Zen fitted well with the military values of the samurai, who used its principles and practices to improve their fighting skills and to learn to accept with equanimity the death that awaited them in battle.

Even in modern Japan, Zen has a close association with the fighting arts of the samurai, kyudo (archery), and kendo (fencing). While the samurai of medieval Japan used Zen to perfect their killing techniques, now it is Zen that uses traditional Japanese archery, stripped of its martial applications, to bring its students to a better understanding of spiritual principles. The ritual of firing the arrow is a form of moving meditation that has little to do with hitting the small target at the end of the firing range.

To the Western mind, which makes a strict division between mind and body, the idea of using a physical discipline to attain spiritual development is an alien one. The main form of motivation for Western athletes is direct competition against other athletes or the ambition to break a world record. Western athletes only recently recognized the mental impact that exercise has on its practitioners, and this impact is still largely ignored except by top athletes who understand the importance of mental training.

Mental training is not just of value to professional athletes but to all of us. Research into the mind-body link reveals that there is a constant interplay between the physical, bio-chemical, and mental levels that impact our well-being. A simple example is the reduced resistance to the common cold that is observed in someone who is recently bereaved. The interaction need not be a purely negative one, however. Doctors are now discovering the chemical basis for the health-giving properties of a "positive attitude."

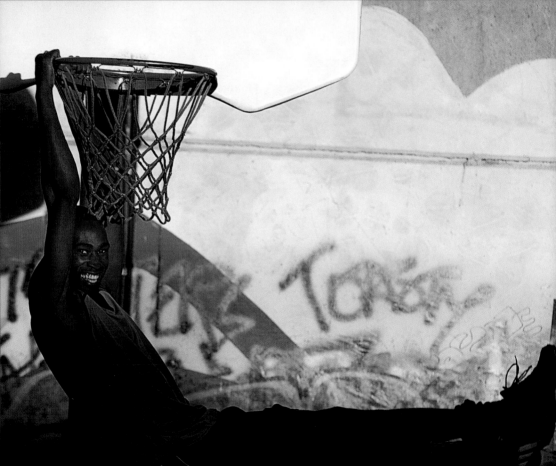

meditating on well-being

This book is divided into eight meditations, each taking one or more aspects of well-being as its theme. This division is necessary for organizational purposes, but somewhat arbitrary, because it is not possible to isolate the overlapping processes of the mind and body that have an effect on well-being.

The first meditation, Right Understanding, examines the past evolution of our mind and bodies, and how this affects our well-being in the present. Three of the meditations—Four, Five, and Six—deal with the physical components of well-being as they are divided by Western fitness culture: flexibility, stamina, and strength. Meditations Two and Three address the question of alternative exercise and therapies and posture; Meditation Seven examines diet and self-image; and Meditation Eight discusses the effects of stress.

Each meditation is followed by a practical section that introduces a variety of techniques and advice in the area under discussion. The examples of workouts and exercises are principally for illustrative purposes—to give the reader a flavor of the techniques—not as courses in the disciplines that require study with an expert teacher.

Just as it is impossible to give advice about lifestyle choices, it is extremely difficult to give practical advice as to the type and frequency of exercises for the mind and body to develop and maintain well-being. It would be impossible to create a single set of recommendations to suit both sexes, and all ages and levels of fitness.

The most important thing that Zen can teach us is how to restore the balance in our lives to attain well-being. This balance should be both within the activities (in strength training, for example, one should perform exercises for all the body's muscle groups, rather than focusing on a select few) and between activities (to devote an equal share of time to the major components of physical and mental well-being).

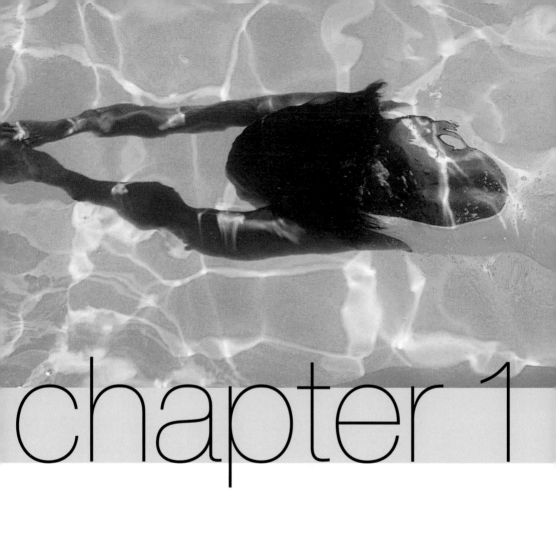

chapter 1

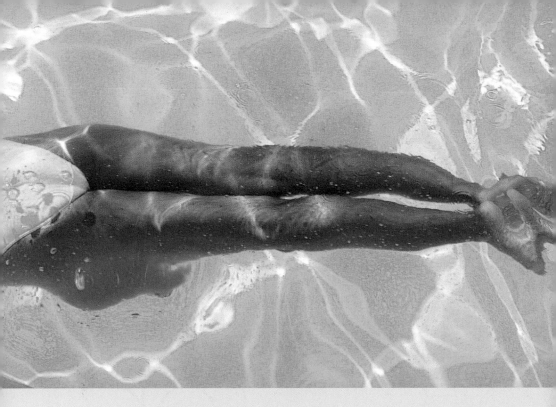

right understanding: physiology

Meditation: "A man's a man for a' that."—Robert Burns

If we are to understand well-being, we first have to look into the distant past of our species. It took homo sapiens four thousand generations to abandon the nomadic, hunter-gathering lifestyle and settle in permanent homes, sow crops, and tame animals, but just four hundred years to invent the computer and send a man to the moon. For 150,000 years our interaction with the natural environment shaped our bodies and brains, but the history of the last five thousand years has shown that we are no longer limited by it. We are now more than the sum of our genetic inheritance, and the consciousness that makes us human gives us a freedom of choice that we can use for our own good or our own destruction.

meet the flintstones

Imagine that you have traveled back into the prehistory of modern humanity, arriving at any time between 150,000 and 10,000 years ago. Wherever you are on the planet, you will encounter small bands of hunter-gatherers. A few cultures close to extinction in the most isolated and inhospitable parts of the world—the South African Bushmen, the "Stone-age" tribes of Papua New-Guinea, the Arctic Inuit, and the Australian Aborigines—are all that survive of this once universal lifestyle.

A study of their lifestyles can give us some idea of how our own distant ancestors lived. This is of more than a passing historical or anthropological interest, because physiologically we are identical to the first humans. And if we want to lead healthy, fulfilled lives, we have to understand exactly how the natural environment shaped our bodies and minds.

Imagine that you have joined one of these nomadic bands in a world where there are no more than a few million humans, and the most advanced technological artifact is the flint axe and the fire-hardened wooden spear. As a hunter-gatherer, you exploit the available resources in the environment—the seasonal harvests of wild fruits, seeds, and roots, and animal prey—but you do not attempt to manipulate the food supply by planting crops or herding animals.

This is not because you do not have the intelligence or the material culture to do so, but because whatever combination of factors made our ancestors settle down—climate change, population pressure, or technological innovation—has not yet taken place. You live in a sophisticated culture, not unlike that of the Plains American Indians, who were hunter-gatherers in a symbiotic relationship with the buffalo until the colonization of North America by European settlers.

You move lightly across the face of the earth. When the seasons turn or the resources of an area are exhausted, you move on, leaving few traces of your passage. Unlike the Flintstones and the Rubbles of cartoon prehistory, you do not have permanent homes. Because you do not control your food supply, you must follow it. Unlike the Plains Indians, however, you have not yet domesticated the horse, so your possessions are limited to what you can carry on your back. You find shelter in natural caves, or build temporary shelters from the available materials you find. During your endless migrations you may be walking twenty miles a day, and even when you have stopped in a place where food is plentiful, there is little time for leisure, as you will spend most of your days engaged in the arduous task of collecting and preparing food.

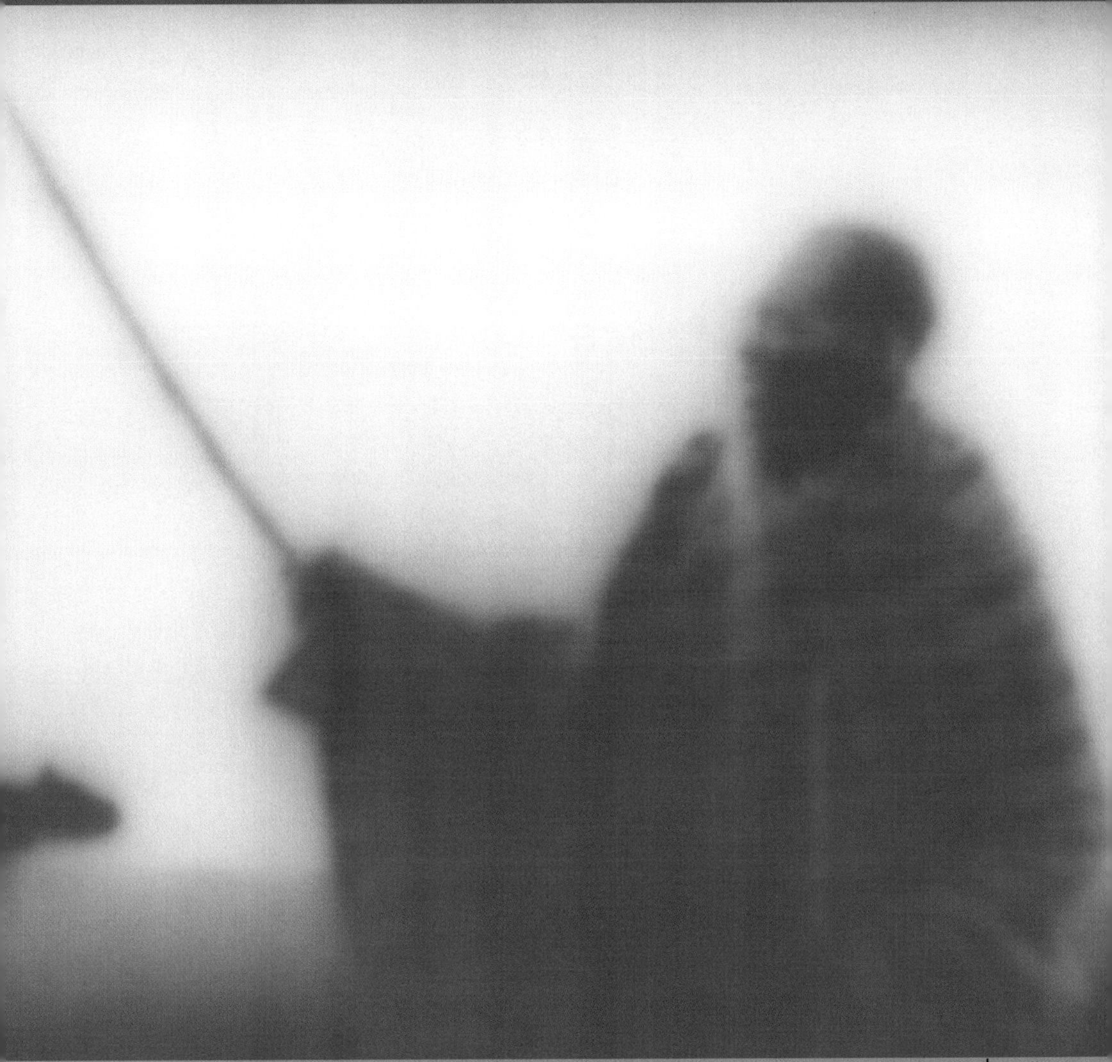

craving calories

The sun rises over a broad valley bounded by high cliffs. You have spent the night sheltering in the relative safety of a natural cave in the cliff face. If you are a healthy male or female adult, you will spend the day hunting among the great herds of herbivores that are the ancestors of our domesticated cattle and horses, and that provide your main source of protein. If you are too young, too aged, a nursing mother, or pregnant, you will spend the day foraging for edible grubs, digging for roots, harvesting seeds, and picking berries and fruit. You stay in a group for safety, always on the look out for predators—lions, bears, wolves—which may snatch the weak or the unwary. The division of labor is not based on any perception of gender inequality but simply because it is difficult to run down an animal when you are too old, pregnant, or have a baby strapped to your back.

In times of scarcity, you may spend the whole day foraging and still may not find enough food to sustain the group. Even in times of plenty, because you do not have the technology to preserve and store food, you must spend most of your day searching for it. The easiest to find—roots, fruits, and berries—is low in calories, and will not sustain you for long. Meat is the most desirable food. It is rich in calories from protein and fat, but requires your hunters to expend a great number of calories in hunting and transporting the carcass back to the band, not to mention the risk of injury during the hunt itself.

Occasionally, your band will find a treat: the honeycomb of wild bees, the sweetest substance found in nature, which will be a flavor feast for your senses and a calorie feast for your body. But for part of the year, at least, you are losing the calorie war, living on the verge of starvation. In this environment, natural selection favors those who have the ability to store the most fuel and preserve it in the form of fat deposits under the skin. This physiology of scarcity has created a highly efficient carbohydrate-fueled musculature, powered by an energy system adapted to long periods of light to moderate exercise, such as walking.

fight or flight

Now imagine that you are in the hunting party, following a herd of herbivores. You know that you and your fellows are not the only hunters stalking the herd. You have rivals—lions, wolves, and hyenas—who will attack you given the opportunity, turning hunter into prey. The hunt exposes you to an incredible amount of mental stress. If you are faced with danger, your instant reaction, mediated by the hormone epinephrine, will be the "fight or flight" response that increases your heartbeat and diverts blood to the limbs.

A lioness threatens a member of the hunting party who has become separated from the group. You feel your pulse race as your realize the danger, your breath becomes shallower, your stomach "knots," and you begin to sweat. You and your fellows act immediately, converging on the lone hunter at full speed, brandishing your stone-tipped spear and uttering fearful war cries. Cowed, the lioness retreats, and your body chemistry slowly returns to normal. It is close to sunset when you return with the carcass of an antelope—the band will feast tonight. For the past few days you have returned empty handed and have had to make do with the harvest of grubs, berries, and fruit gathered by the women. You were growing weaker, and less likely to succeed in capturing a large prey, but the beast was lame and you managed to run it down. You ate some of the meat on the spot, to give yourself the strength to carry the butchered carcass the many miles back to camp. On the way back you have had to fight off other predators and scavengers that wanted to steal your prize.

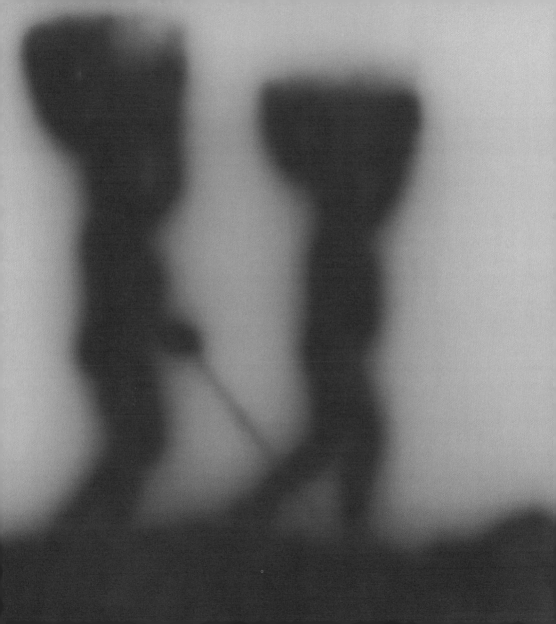

a robust system

If you have stayed behind at the camp, you greet the returning hunters with shouts and ululations of triumph, all anxiety for their safe return forgotten. The fire is built up in the cave as the shadows close in, creating a bright, safe world within. No one will stray outside on his or her own—the world is dangerous and many predators roam the night. Tonight you have forgotten your fears of the dark, and your anxiety about whether you will have enough food. You gorge yourself on roasted meat. The fattiest part of the beast, which is the most highly prized, is given to the hunters.

Your diet of natural, unprocessed, whole foods is alive with bacterial pathogens, but what has not killed you has given you a more robust immune system. You do not have to worry about what you eat. You will never have enough food to become fat. Neither are you at risk from carcinogens or cholesterol, because you will not live long enough to develop either cancer or heart disease.

emotional ties

After
the meal, the lead hunter,
who is the closest person the band has
to a chief, gets up and tells the story of the day's
hunt. You listen in awe to the mighty deeds of each
hunter who brought the beast down; the dangers they
faced to kill the prey and defend it from the scavengers who
wanted to steal it from them. You give thanks to your totem—
the guardian spirit of your band who has brought you this
bounty. You will dance and sing for the spirit, and look at the
mysterious pictures of animals that the chief has painted on
the cave walls.
When the moon is full in the sky, you go to sleep
surrounded by the other members of your band, kept
warm by the heat from their bodies. There is
never a moment in the day or night when
you are alone, and the idea that
you could

ever
be lonely would strike you as
absurd. In this world, it is too dangerous
to remain alone for any length of time.
Social cooperation based on emotional bonding
is the main strategy that allows you and your kind not just
to survive but to thrive in a hostile environment. You will fall in
love, mate, and give birth in full view of your fellows. Despite
the absence of pollution and Genetically Modified Organisms
(GMOs), physical stress, disease, and poor diet mean that you
are old at the age of thirty. When you die, it will be in the arms
of your closest kin, comforted by your belief in a life after
death. When you are buried in a pit in the place where you
died, your body will be arranged in the fetal position,
as if awaiting rebirth. Your few personal effects
will be buried with you, to help you
through the journey in the
afterlife.

back to the future

With considerable relief (especially if you are thirty years of age or older), you are transported back to the present, to the privileged, developed world, where your life expectancy has instantly more than doubled. Long life is not the only difference between your life in the present and the lives of your ancient ancestors. You live a sedentary existence in a permanent home, which is cooled in the summer and heated in the winter. This eliminates a great deal of the physical stress on your body, which will be immediately apparent in your general health and youthful appearance.

With modern conveniences and the mechanization of manual jobs, there is almost no need for any extended physical exertion. You neither have to transport yourself nor your possessions solely by your physical strength—unless it is to lift bags of groceries from the supermarket shopping cart to the trunk of your car, or pick up your suitcase from the airport carousel. Even if you work in a job described as "manual labor," you probably have so many machines at your disposal that you do not expend many more calories than does an office worker.

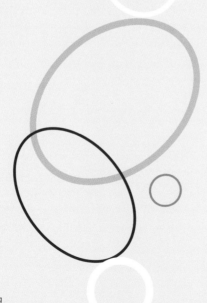

counting calories

If you want to be physically active, you have to make a special effort to add activity into your lifestyle. You may decide to abandon your car and cycle or walk to work, you might develop a taste for gardening or home improvements, or you may choose the more direct route of taking up a sport, going to a gym, or jogging in your leisure time.

If you are not interested in exercise, as your grow older your inactivity will gradually affect your other physical capabilities, such as your hand-eye coordination, balance, strength, posture, the speed of your reflexes, and the range of motion of your joints. But it has the greatest impact on your daily calorie requirements. With an energy system designed for scarcity, you are plunged into a world of calorie excess.

Your body is conditioned to find fatty and sweet foods irresistibly attractive, but you do not have to kill an animal or climb a tree to steal honey from a hive to satisfy your cravings. You merely have to go to the shelf of the closest convenience store; or if you are too lazy even to do that, order over the phone or on-line to have it delivered to your door. Like half the population of the developed world, you are overweight and spend some time in your life attempting to control your weight through limiting the amount of food you eat. Although dieting is only one contributory factor in "eating disorders," it is symptomatic of a loss of balance in our culture's relationship with food.

Despite the enormous variety of food at your disposal, what you eat has never been worse from a health point of view. If you are a North American or Western European, your daily intake contains too much sugar, salt, and fat, as well as many artificial food additives. In addition to the disease-causing agents in your food, you are exposed to dangerous levels of toxins from environmental pollution and smoking.

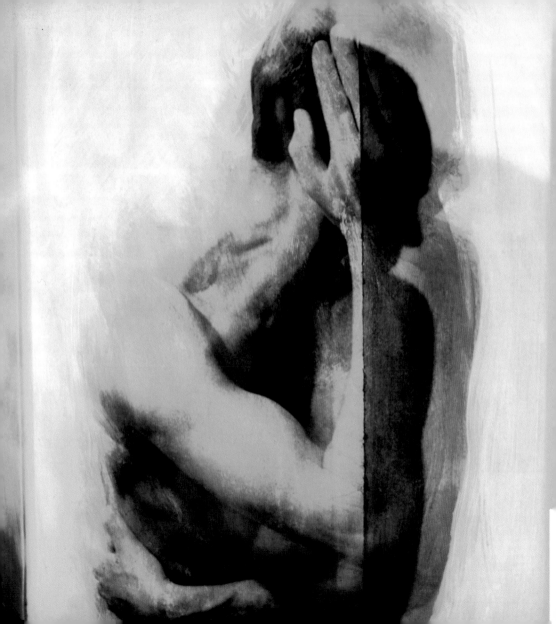

nowhere to run

One of the major risk factors in your lifestyle is stress. Unlike our ancestors whose stress was created by immediate physical threats to which they responded with the fight or flight response, there is no immediate physical release to much of the stress in modern life. Stress from work, relationships, or just the pace of life leads to mental and physical damage throughout the brain and body (see pages 292–293).

One common answer to stress is to seek a chemical solution. You are now more likely than ever to go to ask your doctor for a prescription for tranquilizers or anti-depressant drugs. A significant and growing number of people choose to "self-medicate," using nicotine and alcohol, as well as experimenting with a wide range of illegal substances. Although this may provide temporary relief, and even a limited degree of well-being, it brings with it the many dangers of chemical addiction.

letting the system down

The food in your diet has never been cleaner in terms of bacterial content. But this is a mixed blessing, especially for children and infants. Although they are protected from stomach upsets and minor infections, the absence of bacteria in food and their surroundings means that their immune systems will not kickstart properly, making them more prone to allergies, food intolerances, and other serious illnesses in later life.

loneliness

In a world crowded with seven billion people, you are more likely than ever to spend time on your own—even if you are married and have children. Loneliness caused by social isolation is a major cause of stress, depression, and mental illness. Fears about personal safety and the growth of "anti-social" technologies, such as television and the Internet, leave more and more people fearful and isolated from society.

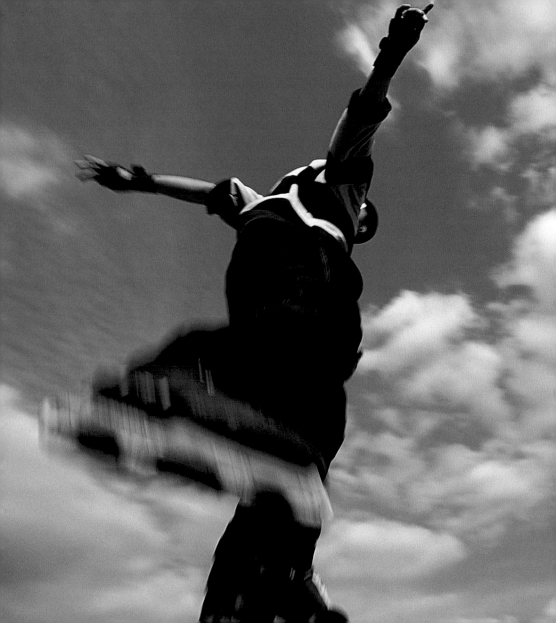

Despite these risk factors, you, along with the other fortunate citizens of the developed world, are the healthiest and oldest humans that have ever lived on the planet. Ironically, you are often the victims of your own success, because it is your longevity that makes you prone to degenerative conditions such as cancer, heart disease, Alzheimer's disease, and arthritis. To borrow from Thomas Hobbes's *Leviathan*: while the lives of your ancestors were "poor, nasty, brutish, and short," yours is more likely to be rich, leisured, lonely, and long.

In our privileged lives, we are all like the historical Buddha, Gautama Siddharta, who was born in a high caste family in India 2,500 years ago. He, too, grew up with all the material advantages available in his day. He lived in the luxury of a palace, where he was never allowed to be bored

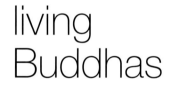

living
Buddhas

or hungry. As a young man he was married to a beautiful woman and fathered a family. The lifestyle that he enjoyed is no longer limited to a tiny ruling elite

In the modern United States and Europe, the majority have the leisure and education to ask the same questions about the meaning of life as the Buddha. In our search for well-being, we are not constrained by time like our ancestors, who had to cram everything into thirty or forty years. The real challenge for modern humans is not mere survival. We have to discover how to live full, happy lives, not just in our twenties and thirties, when we have all the advantages of youth, health, and career success, but into our seventies and eighties.

self-testing

Complete the self-perception index and
compare it with the results of the self-evaluation
on the following pages.

self-perception index (SPI)

This short questionnaire is intended to determine how you perceive your own mental and physical well-being.

Do you feel:

1 Fit

mostly ▢   *sometimes* ▢   *rarely* ▢

2 Active

mostly ▢   *sometimes* ▢   *rarely* ▢

3 Attractive

mostly ▢   *sometimes* ▢   *rarely* ▢

4 Happy

mostly ▢   *sometimes* ▢   *rarely* ▢

5 Healthy

Mostly ▢   *sometimes* ▢   *rarely* ▢

6 Relaxed

mostly ▢   *sometimes* ▢   *rarely* ▢

7 Optimistic

mostly ▢   *sometimes* ▢   *rarely* ▢

8 Successful

mostly ▢   *sometimes* ▢   *rarely* ▢

9 Self-confident

mostly ▢   *sometimes* ▢   *rarely* ▢

self-testing

Complete the questionnaire on the following pages and compare the results with your self-perception index.

self-evaluation

The following self-evaluation consists of simple questions and self-tests that will allow you to evaluate your physical, biochemical, and mental well-being.

There are no "trick" questions; it is obvious in most cases what the "best" answer would be. The questionnaire, however, is not a competition between yourself and others (or some ideal you are trying to live up to). Give yourself an honest evaluation of where you are at the present time with regard to risk factors that affect your well-being.

Once you have completed the questions and self-tests, and refer to page 59 for an analysis of your results. You can use the same questionnaire to monitor future progress.

physical

1) How long do you walk in an average day?

▢ *60 minutes or more*   ▢ *15–55 minutes*   ▢ *less than 15 minutes*

2) How often do you exercise or play a sport per week?

▢ *3 times or more*   ▢ *1–2 times*   ▢ *never*

3) How many push-ups can you do in 1 minute?

▢ *20 or more*   ▢ *5–20*   ▢ *5 or fewer*

4) How long can you remain in an abdominal crunch?

▢ *1 minute or more*   ▢ *30–50 seconds*   ▢ *20 seconds or fewer*

5) From a seated position with your legs straight in front of you, how far can you reach?

▢ *ankles*   ▢ *knees*   ▢ *thighs*

6) Placing your right arm over the back of your head and your left arm behind your back, try and link fingers. How far apart are your fingers? (Repeat with left hand on top and use the average of both for the final result.)

▢ *they interlock*   ▢ *they touch*   ▢ *they are more than 3" apart*

7) Take your pulse for one minute at rest. What is your pulse?

▨ *60 bpm or less* ▨ *60–84 bpm* ▨ *85 bpm or more*

8) After stepping up at a steady speed with an up-up, down-down pattern (right foot up, left foot up, right foot down, left foot down) for three minutes, are you:

▨ *breathing easily* ▨ *breathing heavily* ▨ *breathless*

9) From a standing position, put your right foot as high on your left leg as you can. Put your palms together at chest height and close your eyes. How long can you hold the position? (Repeat with your left foot against your right and use the average of both for the final result.)

▨ *30 seconds or more* ▨ *5–30 seconds* ▨ *5 seconds or fewer*

10) Using a tennis ball or baseball, throw the ball from one hand to the other, and clap your hands in between. Did you succeed:

▨ *on the first try* ▨ *within three tries* ▨ *after more than three tries*

11) Sit in a chair and balance a book on the crown of your head. Slowly rise. Did you succeed:

▨ *on the first try* ▨ *within three tries* ▨ *after more than three tries*

biochemical

12) Is there a history of the following in your family?

- cancer
- heart disease
- arthritis
- diabetes

13) Do you smoke?

- never
- occasionally
- regularly

14) Do you drink alcohol?

- never
- occasionally
- regularly

15) Do you take recreational drugs?

- never
- occasionally
- regularly

16) On average how often do you consult a doctor?

- once a month or more
- at least once a year
- almost never

17) Are you careful about how many calories you eat?

- always
- sometimes
- never

18) Are you careful about how many fat grams you eat?

- always
- sometimes
- never

19) Do you eat five portions of fresh fruit and vegetables every day?

- always
- sometimes
- never

20) If you pinch your waistline can you pinch:

- more than an inch
- about an inch
- less than an inch

mental

21) Are you:

☐ *employed* ☐ *homemaker* ☐ *unemployed*

22) Are you:

☐ *partnered* ☐ *widowed/separated* ☐ *never partnered*

23) On average how often do you laugh in one hour?

☐ *more than three times* ☐ *two–three times* ☐ *once or never*

24) How often do you feel sad or depressed in one day?

☐ *regularly* ☐ *occasionally* ☐ *rarely*

25) Does your job leave you:

☐ *fulfilled* ☐ *indifferent* ☐ *bored*

26) Do you suffer from the following:

☐ *insomnia* ☐ *panic attacks* ☐ *depression* ☐ *food intolerance*

27) Do you think of death?

☐ *often* ☐ *sometimes* ☐ *never*

28) Do you feel valued at home and/or work?

☐ *mostly* ☐ *sometimes* ☐ *rarely*

29) How often do you see friends/socialize in an average week?

☐ *more than three times* ☐ *1–2 times* ☐ *once or never*

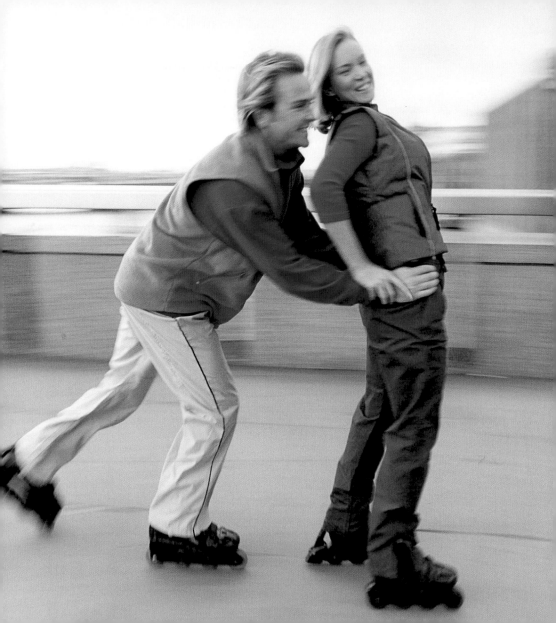

results

Each reply is color-graded. Count how many boxes you have in each color and refer to the analysis below. For a more detailed analysis of the questionnaire, you can analyze your results by subsection:

RED If you have a majority of red boxes, your well-being is being adversely affected by the lifestyle choices you have made. Look through the questions to see if one area needs more attention than the others, and refer to the practical sections of the meditations for advice.

BLUE If you have a majority of blue boxes, you are at a midway point in terms of risk factors in your environment and lifestyle. You have less to do than someone scoring highly in the red zone, but this result is a warning that you need to pay closer attention to certain areas of your life. Check through the questionnaire for areas that need particular attention, and refer to the practical sections of the meditations for advice on how to alter your lifestyle.

YELLOW If you have a majority of yellow boxes, you have reduced the risk factors in your environment and lifestyle and are maximizing your chances to achieve well-being. However, you may have scored in yellow in two out of the three areas, so check the spread of your answers to see if one area still needs attention and refer to the practical sections of the meditations for advice.

Comparison of Self-Perception Index (SPI) and Self-Evaluation

Compare the results from the two questionnaires. If your results match, then you have a realistic view of your own level of well-being. If they are different, you should review the questionnaire to determine the cause of the discrepancy.

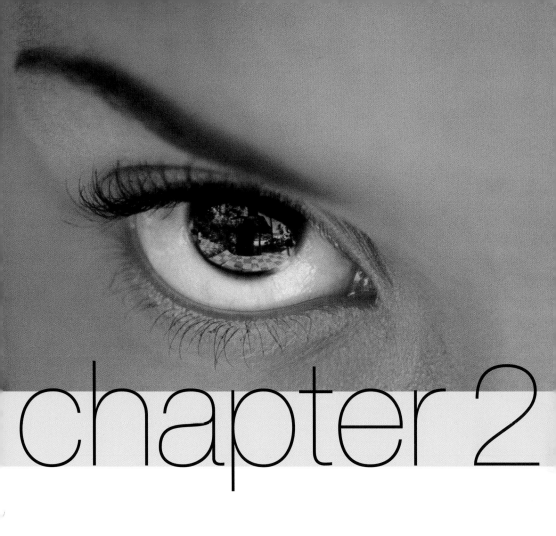

chapter 2

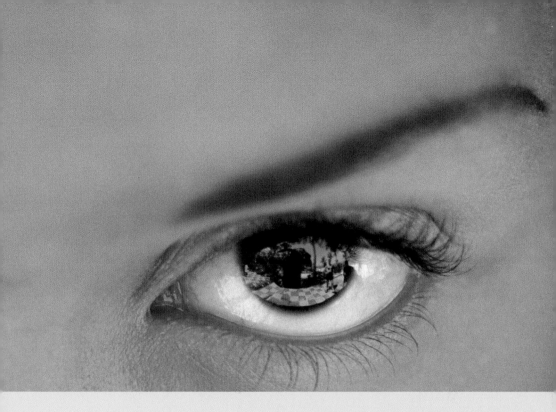

right thought: belief

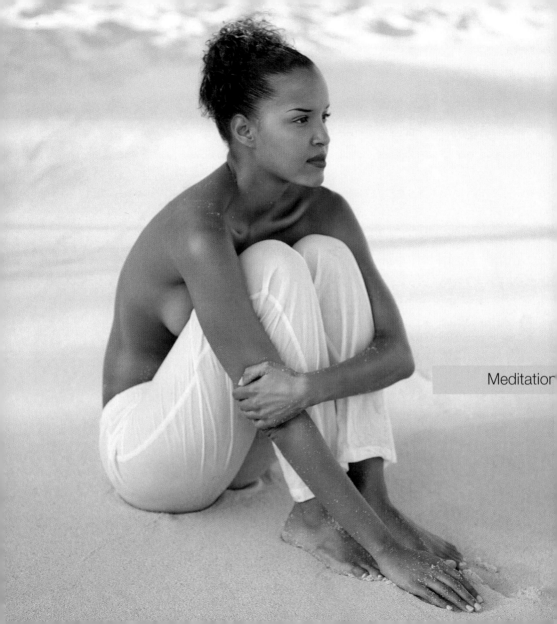

Meditation

undamentally the marksman aims at himself."—*Zen and the Art of Archery*

We would all dearly love to believe in a "magic bullet" that will cure all our physical and mental ills and guarantee us complete well-being. Most still expect that this will be discovered by scientific research, especially now that the Human Genome Project has come to fruition, and we stand on the threshold of a brave new genetic age. For a growing number of people, however, the path to well-being is found in the holistic theories of alternative therapies and exercise systems.

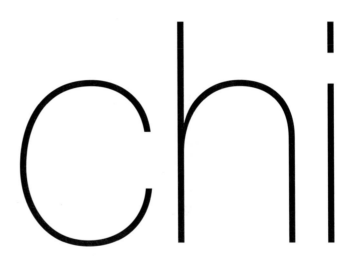

Chi (pronounced chee, and also written qi in the second, more recent, romanization of Chinese) is the central concept that underpins Chinese natural philosophy and medicine. The word is usually translated into English as "energy." However, according to Ted J. Kaptchuk, the first practitioner of traditional Chinese medicine to be employed at a major American hospital, "Chi is not some primordial, immutable material, nor is it merely vital energy [....] Chinese thought does not distinguish between matter and energy, but we can perhaps think of chi as matter on the verge of becoming energy, or energy at the point of materializing." In any case, he adds, the Chinese are not interested in an exact scientific definition of chi but to observe and understand its functions in the universe—that is, to find out what it does.

yin
yang

According to the *Nei Jing* (*The Yellow Emperor's Classic of Internal Medicine*), the earliest Chinese medical text and the foundation of traditional Chinese medicine, chi is composed of the two elemental qualities of yin and yang. Yin, which originally meant "the shady side of the hill," is associated with darkness, cold, damp, stillness, and contraction; yang, originally "the sunny side of a hill," is associated with light, heat, dryness, action, and expansion.

These concepts should not be understood merely as opposites but as complimentary functions, like the two sides of a coin. They are represented in the *t'ai chi* (supreme ultimate) diagram (above right) as a circle divided into two halves—one white and one black—each of which contains the seed of its opposite. Yin and yang exist in a dynamic balance, and when one side becomes dominant, it triggers a transformation that brings its opposite to prominence. It is this interplay that creates and sustains all life in the universe.

harnessing chi

Chi flows around the body through 14 meridians or channels—six on the left side and six on the right. Six of these are yin, and the other six are yang, while the remaining two are the "governing meridians"—one for yin and one for yang.

Unlike Western doctors, who look for the organic causes of disease, such as localized trauma or disease agents (toxins, bacteria, viruses, etc.), traditional Chinese medicine practitioners believe that ill health of the mind and body is due to interruptions or imbalances in the circulation of chi. The treatments they prescribe are "holistic" (i.e., treating the whole person).

In addition to treating the specific symptoms of the disease (like a Western doctor), Chinese doctors aim to re-balance the entire organism. Their treatments include:

- herbal remedies (some of which are now known to be very potent chemically)
- acupuncture
- moxa (burning herbs)
- cupping, or pressure to a selection of the 365 points on the meridians at which chi is concentrated and can enter or leave the body
- dietary advice
- exercise, including *t'ai chi ch'uan* and *chi kung* (or *qigong*, working with energy)

the martial arts

"The warrior must only take care that his

spirit is never broken." —*Shissai*

How these essentially peaceful medical practices became associated with the martial arts is not known. In ancient China, much of the population was not allowed to bear arms, and various forms of unarmed combat developed, which are known in the West under the generic name of kung fu. There are two main styles of unarmed martial arts: hard and soft, or "internal" and "external," which refers to the role of chi in the technique. In the hard martial arts—such as the karate of Japan or the fighting styles demonstrated by Bruce Lee in his many movies—muscular force combined with chi is used to deliver a blow. In the soft martial arts, such as *t'ai chi ch'uan*, chi alone—one's own and the opponent's—is used.

chi kung

If chi can be manipulated to cure illness, the ancient Chinese reasoned, then its store could be increased to prevent it, and maybe even to prolong life.

Over the centuries,
doctors developed exercises
specifically to manipulate chi, and there
is evidence from ancient Chinese tombs of
chi kung dating back 2,500 years. Chi kung
(see page 96) are single movements or
sequences of movements designed to manipulate
an individual's chi. Like Western calisthenics, chi
kung develops a certain degree of flexibility,
stamina, and strength, but these benefits are
considered secondary to the main focus
of the mind, which is on the chi.

Of the several stories explaining the origins of *t'ai chi*, the most fantastic credits its invention to the Taoist monk Chang San-feng, who studied at the Shaolin Temple during the Yuan period (1279-1368). In an interesting aside, the Shaolin tradition of martial arts is said to have been started by the Indian monk Bodhidharma (470-534), the first patriarch of Chinese Zen (Ch'an), who created the exercises to improve the fitness of the monks and allow them to meditate for longer periods. The most likely explanation of the origins of *t'ai chi*, however, is that it developed from a form of hard boxing in the Honan Province during the Ch'ing dynasty (1644-1911). The style was popularized by China's greatest *t'ai chi* master, Yang Lu-ch'an (1795-1872). When Yang was working as a servant, his master, a well-to-do apothecary, engaged a private teacher to initiate his sons into the secrets of *t'ai chi*. Yang spied on the classes through a gap in the garden fence where his master's sons were practicing. He became so expert that he was accepted as a student in his own right. Later he went to Beijing, where he taught the martial arts and famously defeated all comers in boxing competitions. He founded the Yang lineage, passing on his art to his two sons.

Although there are five main styles of *t'ai chi*, Westerners are more likely to encounter the Yang style. In 1956, the Communist authorities created the Beijing Form based on the Yang style. Although traditional *t'ai chi* styles were suppressed during the Chinese Cultural Revolution (1966-69), they have enjoyed a renaissance since the 1980s. The Beijing form is now used by millions of Chinese as a gentle morning fitness routine.

t'ai chi ch'uan

killing the opponent

Many Western teachers of *t'ai chi* promote it as a relaxing and health-promoting exercise and a form of "moving meditation" that deepens consciousness. *T'ai chi*, however, is first and foremost a martial art, the aim of which is the more efficient disabling, and if necessary, killing of one's opponent.

There is nothing intrinsically moral or good about t'ai chi or its associated practices. A simple analogy would be that chi, like electricity, can be good or bad— good when it lights a lamp, bad, when it electrocutes someone. A cursory look through the biographies of the great t'ai chi masters of the past reveals that they were not holy sages spreading enlightenment, but often womanizers, drinkers, and tavern brawlers, who sold their skills to the highest bidder. Interestingly, there are no women masters of *t'ai chi* in Chinese tradition.

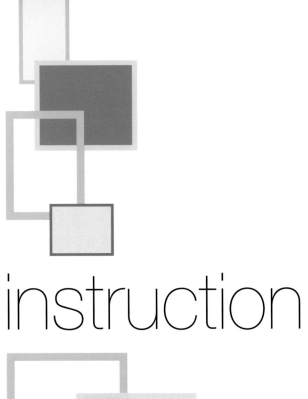

instruction

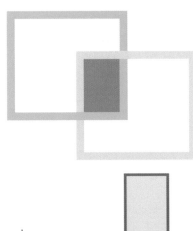

When you join a *t'ai chi* class, you may wish to approach its study from two very distinct perspectives: you may simply wish to learn a new form of exercise, or you can embark on the study of a new philosophy that will affect every aspect of your lifestyle. The teaching method you will encounter is entirely different from what you are used to in a yoga or aerobics class. When you learn a Western sport or fitness technique, for example, the coach or teacher will start with a lecture on theory. In a t'ai chi class, there is little talking, save for basic instructions, and no explanations of theory. T'ai chi teachers follow the Chinese method of instruction: the teacher demonstrates and the pupil copies until he or she masters the exercise. Then you move on to the next exercise.

Teachers teach this way because that is how they were taught themselves, and because they know that an explanation would be useless, especially when what is being learned can only be performed and felt. This is in itself beneficial to Westerners who feel they must always know why they are doing something. In a t'ai chi class, the teacher is king. You can obey his instructions, or you can leave.

An average 90-minute to 2-hour class begins with a warm-up (see page 95), followed by chi kung exercises (see page 96). Both stimulate and balance the flow of chi. With the chi activated and, coincidentally, the joints and muscles thoroughly warmed up just as they would be by a standard warm-up with movement and stretches, the teacher will then lead his class through other exercises, such as t'ai chi walking (see page 98–99).

In addition to illuminating various aspects of the technique, these are a stealthy way to introduce strengthening exercises to students who have never done a push-up or lifted a weight in their lives. In good Karate Kid fashion, the wily instructor instructs his pupil to "paint the fence" and "polish the car" in very specific ways. The repetition of simple actions not only strengthens the muscles and joints, but also teaches the body patterns that it will later perform instinctively without recourse to the conscious mind.

Although one cannot see the process in oneself, you can easily observe it in beginners who come after you in the class; they will unconsciously progress from the ungainly, uncoordinated steps of their first efforts, to smooth, flowing movements in a matter of weeks.

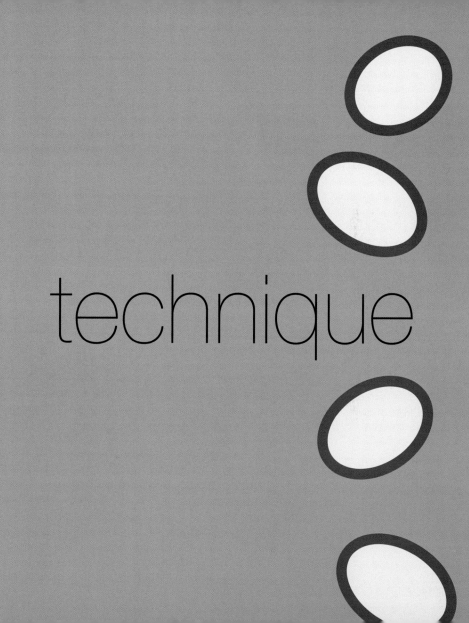

technique

The main component of a *t'ai chi ch'uan* class is the form, which consists of between twenty-four movements (Beijing form) to well over one hundred movements (Long Yang Form) in a flowing sequence. Depending on how much practice a student is willing to put in, the basic movements of the form can be mastered in three to six months.

Performed competently, the form seems an effortless slow-motion dance. But even for someone with above-average physical fitness, it is a demanding exercise that develops coordination, balance, endurance, and strength, as well as mental control. The process is slow and steady, and students are only dimly aware of the gains they are making with each class. The form is only one of the tools t'ai chi uses to train the mind and body.

form

Once they are able to perform the full sequence, students feel a great sense of accomplishment and satisfaction. But this is only the beginning. The performance of the form can always be improved and refined, and there are several forms in each style, using the sword, spear, and dagger, and pushing hands practice (slow-motion sparring) in which you attempt to "uproot" (unbalance) your partner and make him or her trip.

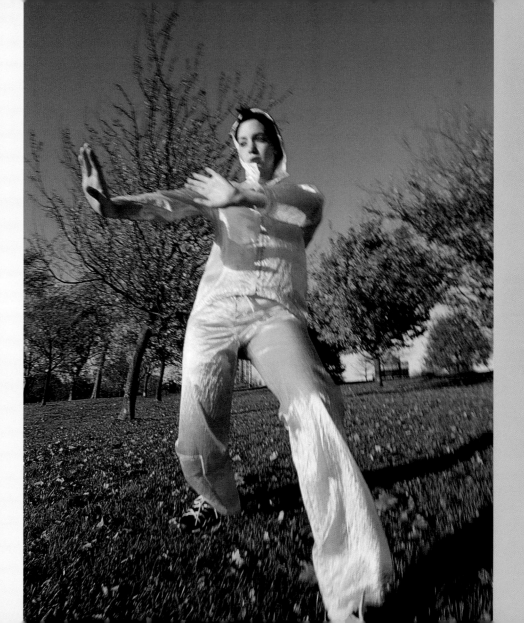

A second outcome of studying *t'ai chi* according to the Chinese method is the group dynamics that develop within the class. The students get something of a "chosen-few" mentality, in that they feel that they are being initiated into esoteric and exotic secrets that outsiders are excluded from. This is partly a form of self-defense, as the uncomprehending glances of onlookers are not always looks of awed, respectful silence.

A well-attended class, with new students joining throughout the year gives the teacher the opportunity to delegate the teaching of beginners to senior students. A hierarchy quickly develops in the top echelons of the class, and students compete with one another to win the teacher's approval and favor. This creates a pool of enthusiastic, unpaid teaching assistants, but this should not be seen as exploitation on the teacher's part, as the process of teaching helps the senior students in their own development.

The Chinese teaching system implies reciprocal obligations, on the part of both teacher and pupil, which far exceed the mere exchange of money that takes place between teacher and student of an aerobics or yoga class. You will be expected to attend the teacher's weekly classes, respect an etiquette of Chinese-style bows, dress code, and behavior, and follow the teacher's advice, which may go beyond health and fitness into areas of your private life. Beyond the class activities, you will be expected to perform your daily practice of the form for twenty to thirty minutes every morning. The most enthusiastic students are so taken up by t'ai chi that it soon affects every aspect of their lives. The most enthusiastic students will become teachers in their own right.

pupil becomes teacher

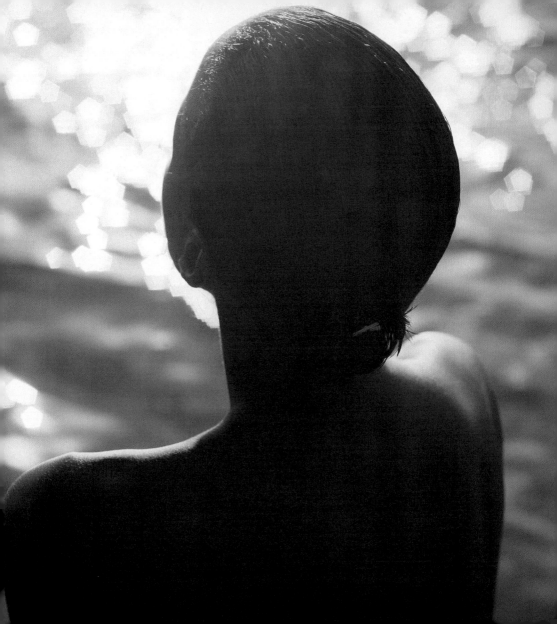

do you believe?

I have explained some of the traditional beliefs on which *t'ai chi* is based, which are finding increasing acceptance in the Western world. In tandem with the growing popularity of *t'ai chi* and other Chinese martial arts, people flock to clinics offering traditional Chinese medicine treatments such as acupuncture and Chinese herbs. And feng-shui, the art of manipulating chi in the environment to improve one's health and good fortune, is transforming Western interior design. Once skeptical, scientific-minded Westerners now put their faith in traditional Chinese wisdom. But what evidence, if any, has been gathered so far to validate these beliefs?

In China itself, traditional Chinese medicine all but disappeared in the major cities with the introduction of Western medicine after the advent of the Chinese republic 1911–49. It was only after the Maoist revolution that the Communist regime, chronically short of trained medical personnel, turned to it to fill the gap, training thousands of "barefoot doctors" in herbal medicine and acupuncture to provide inexpensive primary health care and education in rural areas.

In the West, the medical establishment has accepted the notion of holistic medicine, but it remains skeptical as to the specific claims of Chinese doctors. Research has failed to provide proof of the existence of chi or the meridians, and trials of Chinese herbs and acupuncture have shown only limited success in a few conditions, notably in the treatment of eczema and irritable bowel syndrome.

Yet, how do we account for the growing popularity of non-Western and alternative therapies, such as traditional Chinese medicine and Indian Ayurvedic medicine (see page 136)? Their increasing popularity in the parts of the world with the most advanced systems of scientific health care seems to indicate that they provide something that high-tech machines and drugs cannot.

Even if we take into account the benefits of the chemically active ingredients that have been found in herbal medicine from India and China (which act very much like our own synthetic drugs) and the effects of changes in diet and exercise, there is another factor that gives these therapies a unique appeal and an observable degree of effectiveness.

the placebo effect

One likely explanation comes from the work of Dr Herbert Benson of the Mind-Body Institute of the Harvard Medical School. He focuses on the potency of the mind-body link in alternative therapies that is demonstrated by the "placebo effect." Placebo (Latin for "I will please") is a completely inert medicine, like colored water or a sugar pill, given to humor a patient who does not need drug therapy.

In many trials, up to 90 percent of patients dosed with a completely inert substance said that they felt better, and objective tests confirmed that their condition had improved. Results vary depending on the person administering the placebo. A trusted figure, who the patient likes and respects, will produce better results than an unsympathetic person. There is also such a thing as an "anti-placebo effect," in which an otherwise effective treatment fails because the patient is unhappy about the way it is administered.

We know that emotional states have physiological effects. Stress, loneliness, and anxiety, for example, reduce the immune response. Someone undergoing a divorce or bereavement is twice as likely to catch a cold. A positive mental attitude, on the other hand, can assist in both the treatment and recovery from disease. The survival rates of cancer patients increase if they are determined to defeat the disease, or in complete denial. The lowest survival rates are recorded for those who are fatalistic about their lot or feel helpless.

Once the body is seriously compromised, however, as in HIV-AIDS or in the advanced stages of cancer, the mind-body link has little impact. Its effectiveness is limited to minor ailments and preventative care. In this, scientific studies match the theories of chi, for chi is a positive energy that enhances physical health and mental well-being, rather than producing them.

the skeptic's response

For the skeptic, chi can be seen as a prescientific metaphor for physical processes that the ancient Chinese did not understand: the circulation of blood and hormones, the biochemistry of the brain, and the functioning of the nervous system. In traditional belief, chi is seen as the underpinning of all these processes: it enters the body with the air, is transported in the bloodstream, is absorbed with food, and passes into the body.

the believer's response

For believers, *t'ai chi* and *chi kung* are holistic forms of exercise that integrate the mental, biochemical, and physical levels in a set of exercise and lifestyle guidelines, and exploit the mind–body link to increase well-being. Unfortunately, there is no way that the effectiveness of many alternative techniques can be tested by conventional trials. (How could you give placebo acupuncture or placebo *chi kung*?)

story

leap of faith

"Come running at me, arms straight out in front of you, and keep your eyes shut," the teacher instructed. "Are you ready?" he said looking over my shoulder at the two students standing by the wall on the other side of the room. They smiled nervously at him.

I had waited in line with the other members of the class, and now it was my turn. I closed my eyes as ordered and raised by arms to shoulder height. The teacher was about five feet in front of me, standing with his back to the wall, so even with my eyes shut, I was unlikely to miss him. He was about five feet nine inches and did not weigh more than 150 pounds, while I was a good three inches taller and twenty-five pounds heavier, with the muscle mass of a regular weight-trainer. If I ran at full speed as he had ordered me to, I should, by rights, smash him into the wall and make a dent in the plasterwork.

"Don't hold back," he said, as if he was reading my mind.

In the "crash course" in belief our teacher was giving his students about the properties of chi, he had told us that he would use our own chi to bounce us to the back wall. The two students were stationed there to prevent us from hurting ourselves.

I was dimly aware that several things were being tested here: our trust and respect for our teacher were both high on the list. With my eyes shut, time seemed to dilate, and it felt as if it was taking much too long to cross the few feet of bare floorboards that separated us.

Like a bungie-jumper whose elastic band has run out of slack, I reached the teacher. The events that followed happened too fast for me to register them clearly, but I felt the forward momentum of my body somehow being deflected in a downward circular motion. When I opened my eyes, I was on the other side of the room being steadied by the two students instructed to catch me. Stunned, I stared at the teacher, who told me to get out of the way. I was so dazed by the experience that by the time I had recovered the demonstration had finished.

What had happened? The part of me that believes in chi believes that the teacher manipulated my chi in some mysterious way; the skeptic in me thinks that I did it to myself through autosuggestion. I wanted so hard to believe, and the teacher assisted me in setting the scene with dimmed lighting, warnings, and an implanted suggestion of what was about to happen.

The class ended, and the students, silent and pensive went their separate ways. The matter was never brought up again.

t'ai chi
and chi kung guidelines

The slow-paced movements of *t'ai chi* and *chi kung* make them suitable for people with a low degree of physical fitness, older individuals, as well as people returning to exercise after an illness. However, physically fit people will also be challenged by *t'ai chi*, both physically and mentally. In China, *t'ai chi* is studied by martial artists once they have attained a high degree of endurance, flexibility, and strength through learning "hard" styles of boxing.

I have chosen several basic *t'ai chi* and *chi kung* exercises that will give you a flavor of *t'ai chi* practice. However, the only way to experience *t'ai chi* properly is to participate in a class.

warm up

Perform each exercise for thirty seconds to one minute.

- Stand with your feet shoulder width apart; arms by your side, and swing your arms from the shoulders, bending your knees each time your hands swing past them.

- Rotate your trunk from the waist, trying to keep forwrd and your hips square. Do not lead with your shoulders. Increase the pace of the turn, until your hands slap your shoulders. Change the direction of the rotation.

- **Neck circles**

  Slowly rotate your head to the right keeping a constant speed. Reverse the direction of the rotation.

- **Shoulders**

  With your arms hanging loosely by your sides, raise your shoulders as high as you can and roll them forward. Let them drop and roll backward. Reverse the direction of the rotation.

- **Hip circles**

  With your palms on your lower back, make a large circle with your hips. Reverse the direction of the rotation.

- **Knee circles**

  With your hands resting lightly on your thighs and your knees together, make a circle with your knees inward; move slowly and smoothly. Reverse the direction of the rotation.

chi kung: "raising the chi"

- Stand with feet shoulder-width apart, arms easy by your sides. Your head and back are straight, but your chest and shoulders are relaxed. Your knees are straight but not locked. Breathe deeply through your nose, relaxing your stomach muscles and tucking your tailbone in, almost as if you were sitting on a stool. Your mind is held at a point two inches below your navel, the tantien, the body's main chi reservoir, and your body's center of gravity. As you breath in, imagine that you are taking in chi with each breath, directing it into your tantien.

- Once you are breathing evenly and deeply, your mind is quiet, and your body is free of tension, slowly raise your hands, palms facing down. They should float up, as if pulled up by invisible strings. Your arms and shoulders should remain free of tension and relaxed, and your mind focused on your breath and the tantien. Stop your arms when they reach shoulder height. The fingers should point forward, but the finger joints should not be locked.

- Breathe out and soften your shoulders and elbows, allowing your hands to float down. Maintain the same speed throughout the exercise. When your hands reach your hips, bend your knees slightly.

- Straighten and raise your arms as before, but this time raise them a little higher than shoulder height. Keep to the breathing pattern. Continue until your arms are over your head and then lean back as far as is comfortable.

- Breathe out and lower your hands to return to the starting position.

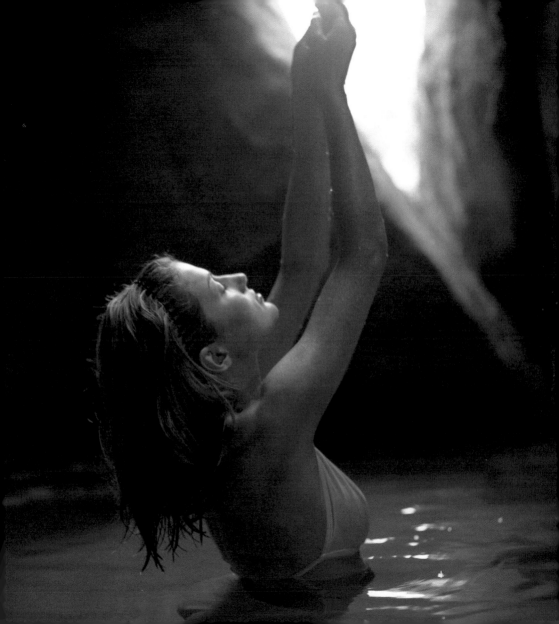

t'ai chi walking "brush knee"

- Stand with your left foot in front of you, toes facing forward, and your back foot turned out at a forty-five-degree angle. Your legs should be bent at the knees and shoulder-width apart; your waist is facing forward with your hips square. Your back and head are straight, but your shoulders and chest are relaxed and sunken (not puffed up). Place your left hand at waist height on the outside of your right left knee, palm facing down, and your right hand at chest height, palm facing forward. The elbows of both arms are soft and rounded.

- Turn your waist toward the left, and sit back on your right leg, so that all your weight is over your right foot. Lift your left toes off the ground and turn them out to the right to forty-five degrees. At the same time let your arms sink. Your left arm will circle back until your left hand is at shoulder height.

- Shift all your weight onto your left foot, and take a step forward with your right foot, toes facing forward. Your feet should remain shoulder-width apart. Turn your waist to the right and "brush" your right knee, so that your right hand ends up on the outside of your knee at waist height, palm down.

- Shift the weight to your right foot, and complete the step by bringing your left hand in front of you, palm facing out at chest height. You are now standing in a mirror image of the starting position. Repeat the movements, stepping from one foot to the other for the length of the room. Keep the movement slow, continuous, and fluid. The idea is to coordinate the action of the arms, legs, and waist.

building leg strength— "playing the lute"

- Stand with all your weight on your bent right leg. Your left leg is in front of you, resting on the heel of the left foot. Make sure that there is no weight on the left leg by lifting it off the floor. Hold your arms in front of you, left arm extended, palm facing right; right arm, bent at the elbow, palm facing the left elbow. Hold for as long as you can, building up to five minutes, then swap sides and repeat, standing in the mirror image of the first posture.

chapter 3

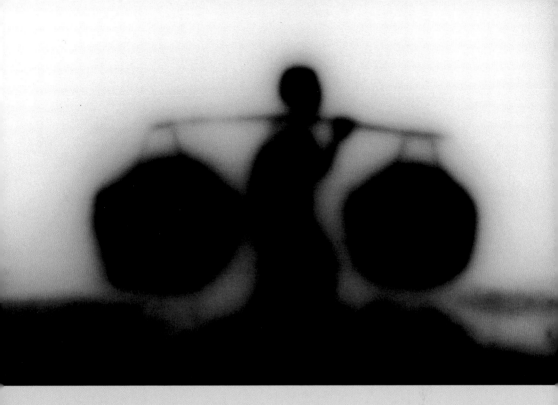

right attention: posture

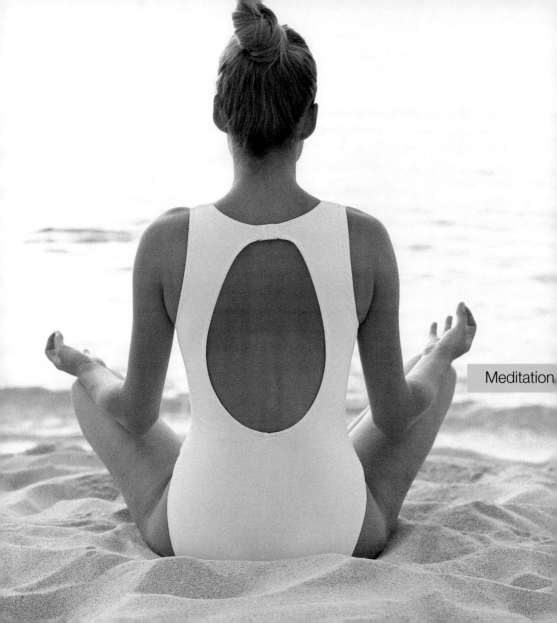

Meditation

n walking, just walk. In sitting, just sit. Above all, don't wobble." —Yun-men

Correct posture—the proper alignment of the skeleton, joints, and musculature, at rest and during movement—is the foundation of physical well-being. Even slight deviation from proper alignment, caused by injury, stress-induced muscle tension, or poor postural habits, can, over decades, lead to physical problems that do not respond to conventional medical treatment. In these circumstances, many increasingly turn to "alternative therapies" for help. But instead of only teaching practical techniques to deal with what are often purely physical problems, many alternative therapists offer belief systems and lifestyle advice.

a failure in western medicine?

At the turn of the twenty-first century, life expectancies of seventy-five years for men and eighty years for women in Western nations are still in marked contrast with the much lower life spans of people in the developing world. With this in mind, it was with some interest that, during the 1980s, I watched the emergence of a multitude of "alternative therapies" in the West. As I was living in Asia at the time, I was in a position to contrast the attitudes of people of the countries where several of these techniques had originated with those of their Western exponents and practitioners. While Westerners claimed that thousands of years of practice and millions of present-day adherents must prove the value of non-Western medical theories and techniques, anyone in Asia who could afford to had long ago opted for Western scientific medicine and were, for the most part, ignorant of their own indigenous traditions.

An important fact that supporters of alternative therapies continue to ignore in their literature is that these therapies originate in countries where life expectancy, infant survival rates, general health, and quality of life are vastly inferior to our own. One non-Western nation which does not have such depressing statistics is Japan, which has the longest life expectancy in the world. This, however, is not due to an alternative view of health and fitness or adherence to non-Western medical practices. Japan not only has an excellent scientific medical infrastructure, its population also has a huge dietary advantage over Europeans and Americans: the Japanese eat a low-fat diet, and they eat in moderation, which results in lower rates of obesity and its many related diseases. While they score highly for avoiding heart disease and many cancers, the Japanese have the highest rates of cancers of the intestinal tract, because of an over-refined diet that is lacking in fiber.

Despite Western medicine's obvious success in treating disease and prolonging life, it is clear that it is also in crisis. The cause is clearly not to be found in failure, so it must lie in its success. Instead of leading "nasty, short, and brutish" lives, punctuated by terrible diseases, we live long and healthy lives until an advanced age when we succumb to degenerative conditions against which twenty-first century medicine has little to offer. The fact that we have contributed to our own conditions through our lifestyle choices—poor diet, lack of exercise, and smoking—make it all the worse.

In the 1990s, when I was working as a health and fitness journalist, I was daily exposed to the claims of alternative therapies of every complexion. Alarmed by the flood of uncritical articles that were appearing almost daily in the print media, I persuaded my editor to commission a series of first-hand accounts of alternative therapies that would debunk the therapies if and when necessary. I was not setting out to attack all alternative therapies, but merely put them into perspective and determine what they could be used for. I ruled out what I felt were the more outlandish therapies—faith healing, reiki, crystal therapy, etc—because it would be too easy to ridicule their claims.

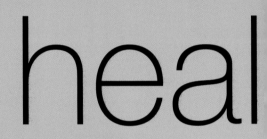

I had already experienced osteopathy and various forms of massage, the former for minor training injuries and the latter for relaxation, but there was one technique that I had long wanted an excuse to try out, the Alexander Technique (AT). Unfortunately, apart from a yearly bout of flu and some minor training injuries, I am plagued with good health. I do, however, like everyone who spends most of the working day seated at a desk, working at a computer, get a sore lower back from time to time, so it was this problem that I took with me to my first Alexander session.

thyself

I turned up for the first of a course of twenty 45-minute lessons at 8 a.m.

My Alexander teacher (note: not therapist), Kieron, was not what I had expected from a New Age therapist. Although not dressed in a medical white coat, his dress sense had nothing alternative about it, nor did his treatment room; there was a distinct absence of incense, mandalas, and ambient whale music—just a table, several straight-back chairs, and medical charts of the human skeleton and musculature on the wall. This was reassuring, but I retained my skepticism for the time being.

"Let's get a couple of things straight before we start," Kieron said. "AT is not about posture, and it isn't an alternative therapy. There's no mumbo jumbo, no special diet, and you don't have to hug anybody."

I was relieved, but my first two preconceptions had been shattered. I tried to sit comfortably on the edge of a straight-backed, wooden chair, and gave him my full attention. Kieron, however, did have all the fire and zeal of the true believer.

"Let's start with posture. Anyone can ram themselves into perfect posture (you draw an imaginary line from your ears, through the shoulders, hips, knees and ankles); but once you're there you're stuck; as soon as you move, you lose the alignment. One of the things AT sets out to teach is poise, that is, to maintain good posture all the time, dynamically."

He went on to explain that the Alexander Technique is not an alternative therapy, because it does not claim to cure anything. But Kieron admitted he was seeing an increasing number of therapeutic referrals—people suffering from neck and back pain, headaches, and other stress-related symptoms. He told them that AT would not deal with their problem directly, but if the condition were stress-related and not mechanical (i.e., an illness or injury), relief of their symptoms would be one of the by-products of learning the technique.

Frederick Alexander

"The choices we make about what we do with ourselves to a large exter

The Alexander Technique was created by a performer at the end of the nineteenth century. Frederick Alexander was a native of the isolated town of Wynward, on the island of Tasmania, Australia. Born in 1869, he grew up as one of eight children on a farm. As a young child, he was taken out of school because of respiratory problems. He continued his education privately and as his health improved, he developed twin passions for horses and the theater. He left home at 16, and worked while he trained as an actor and a musician. In his twenties he became a performer, specializing in monologues. However, his respiratory problems affected his delivery, and on several occasions his voice failed him during a performance.

Doctors were unable to help him, so he took matters into his own hands and searched for a cure. He knew that he had no problems with ordinary speech, only during his public recitations. He started to observe his "manner of doing" while speaking and reciting. As he watched himself in a mirror, he noticed several habitual actions when he started to recite: he stiffened his neck causing his head to go back, he depressed his larynx, and he sucked in breath with a gasp.

Studying himself more closely, he noticed that he also did this in ordinary speech but in a much milder form so that there was no visible effect. The only difference was one of degree. He had discovered what he termed "a pattern of misuse," which he set out to correct. Although he could not consciously do anything about the way he breathed and depressed his larynx, he began by preventing himself from pulling back his head, which slightly improved the other two problems. He concluded that his "manner of doing affected his functioning."

He experimented with head positions, noticing that when he depressed his larynx he also lifted his chest, narrowed his back, and shortened his stature. Alexander now realized that his voice was not only influenced by his head and neck but by the position of his whole body, discovering the crucial relationship between head, neck and torso, which he called "Primary Control." Despite this initial advance, when he looked at himself in the mirror, he realized that, "When I tried to combine the prevention of shortening with a positive attempt to maintain a lengthening and speak at the same time, I did not put my head forward and up as I intended, but actually put it back... I was doing the opposite of what I believed and of what I had decided to do."

The greatest obstacle, he realized, was habit, which was made worse by years of theatrical training. He discovered that what "felt right" was determined by force of habit, and although it was completely wrong, that it was much stronger than his ability to change. Optimistic about his own ability, however, he wrote: "Surely if it is possible for feeling to become untrustworthy as a means of direction, it should also be possible to make it trustworthy again."

He continued to elaborate his methods until his death in 1955. Alexander Technique training begins with "inhibition"—recognizing and stopping a bad habit—followed by conscious "direction," re-training the body into new, better patterns of use. Having cured his own voice problem, he went on to become so celebrated an orator that he attracted pupils as a voice coach. In time, he realized that his method could be applied to improve the performances of all kinds of performers, actors, musicians, and dancers.

Kieron handed me a large lead ball that weighed about eight and a half pounds. It felt very heavy—not something I'd be able to hold at arms' length for long. "This is about a couple of pounds less than the average skull," he told me.

"Your head is balanced on top of a curved spring, made of bones and fluid-filled cartilage disks called the spine, whose job it is to send your head as far away from the ground as possible. Attached all along the spine are a series of tough elastic muscles, which, as well as allowing you to move, are designed to maintain the optimum shape of the spine."

The problem with modern living is that it encourages us to look down all the time: when we drive, eat, when we read, write, or work on a computer, and if taller than average, when we talk to shorter people. This brings the head forward, and as it's extremely heavy, it pulls the back, neck, and shoulders forward and down. The muscles of the back and neck have to be in constant contraction to compensate for the forward position of the head, and over decades, they "learn" that this is their natural position, even when we are standing up and not looking down. In AT, this is known as "residual contraction"—one of the bad patterns of use that Alexander discovered. Instead of holding the spine up and allowing it to do its job, the muscles are actually pulling it out of shape, and the results can be tension headaches, back and neck pain, and in extreme cases, compressed spinal disks. We have literally learned to give ourselves back pain. The AT solution is to "free" the neck and back muscles, allowing the body to remember the best position for the head.

unlearning habit
unlearning habit
unlearning habit
unlearning habit
unlearning habit
unlearning habit
unlearning habit
unlearning habit
unlearning habit
unlearning habit

how it works

The learning process works in two ways, by direct instruction from the teacher, who encourages a repositioning of the body, and by your own analysis of the changes that the teacher is encouraging to take place. In the first session Kieron concentrated on releasing my neck muscles. He held my neck and upper back, and seemed to be doing very little, but 15 minutes into the session, my eyes began to blur, I felt queasy, and my lower back was complaining. I had to have a break. Kieron was apologetic, "I try and avoid this but I've worked you quite hard. It's probably a reaction of the balance organs in the ears. They are used to your head being in one position, and when the neck muscles are released and your head moves into a new position, they get confused and send scrambled signals to your brain. The feeling passes quickly."

So how does it work? "I am standing here," Kieron explained, "ordering my body to do absolutely nothing. There's no magic or psychic transfer of energy. All I've done is put my own body into 'neutral,' that is, I am using the least amount of muscular effort to stand and move. Your body is sensitive enough to tune into that state, and thinks to itself, I want to feel like that too."

"All your body needs is a hint, and it does the rest of it for itself." "The first five sessions are the worst," Keiron said cheerfully. And he was right. During the next three weeks, no position I tried when I was sitting or standing seemed quite right. Muscles that had been in tension for years were releasing, and they were letting me know about it. "If someone comes in with back or neck pain, it usually clears up after the fifth or sixth session," Kieron said, "but that's only the beginning. Then they can learn how to use their bodies properly."

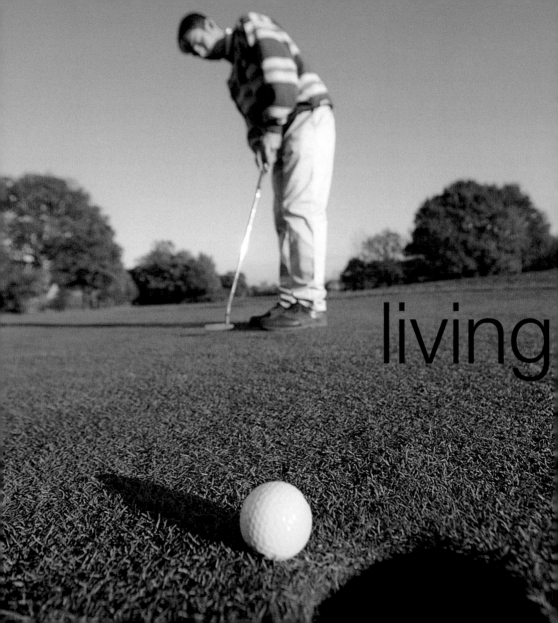

living

I could see myself going into zealot mode. I would start a crusade ridding the world of the evils of the squashy sofa, the comfy chair, and worst of all, cushions—all secret torture instruments designed to lead us astray from postural salvation. "We can't change the world," Kieron said, bringing me back to reality with a jolt. "You have to sit on sofas and be in bad posture for some of the time, but that doesn't mean that you have to carry that bad posture around with you once you stand up."

In subsequent sessions, Kieron worked on the other major joints—shoulders, hips, knees, and ankles. As the tension released, I realized how little I controlled my body over the past decades. "People live in a blur of habit," Kieron said, "using a lot more effort than is necessary to do simple actions like typing or sitting."

in the real world

In the more advanced stages of the technique, students start to notice other less obvious benefits. As tension in the shoulders and chest releases, the ribcage is free to open to full capacity, improving breathing and increasing the oxygen supply to the brain and muscles. They feel more energetic because they are saving large amounts of energy that they used to waste. There are also psychological gains. Kieron explained: "I've seen tall people, who've been trying to make themselves smaller all their lives, literally unfold and straighten up. But students also feel more confident because their bodies are less reactive. They learn not to tense up in stressful situations and to remain poised."

a good technique

The Alexander Technique is a form of therapy that I endorse wholeheartedly. It is circumscribed in its aims and claims. It is not selling you a belief system or a lifestyle, but a technique to apply to specific problems. For it to work, you don't have to believe in it, just as you don't have to believe in aspirin for it to cure your headache. If you are looking for a religion or a new lifestyle, be honest about it. You will not obtain it from an AT teacher, but you will find plenty of others who will accept you and your money with open arms.

general posture guidelines

The Alexander Technique sets out to correct patterns of misuse that you may have acquired over a lifetime in the most basic of actions: standing, sitting, walking, running. Misuse is encouraged by poor postural habits, so analyze your posture with regard to the position of your head and spine.

Pay particular attention to the site of old injuries. We learn to shield injuries to allow them time to heal, but sometimes, even when the original injury is no longer a physical problem, we retain the shielding behavior. In other words, we have adapted to a different pattern of use. This may have no immediate effect on the body, but over a period of twenty years, it may lead to major physical problems.

alleviating back pain

For millions, back pain is an intractable problem that conventional medicine can do little to alleviate. There is no single cause for back pain, but for the majority of people who experience back pain, it is caused by a combination of poor postural habits, insufficient flexibility in the hamstrings, and weaknesses in the abdominal muscles.

Before consulting a conventional or an alternative therapist, you should first attempt a program of self-help. To begin:

- stretch your back on a daily basis (see pages 158–159)
- strengthen your stomach muscles with the mid-body workout given on pages 238–242
- look at your work environment (desk height, etc.) for any potential causes of your problem
- increase your awareness of your body position while sitting, standing, and during everyday tasks, especially all those involving lifting

semi-supine position

This position is recommended for relaxation and realigning the body.

Lie on your back with your head resting on a paperback book (the idea is for the head to be neither tilted back or forward, but in alignment with the spine). Bend your legs at the knees. Keep your feet on the floor and your arms by your sides. Stay in the position for a minimum of twenty minutes.

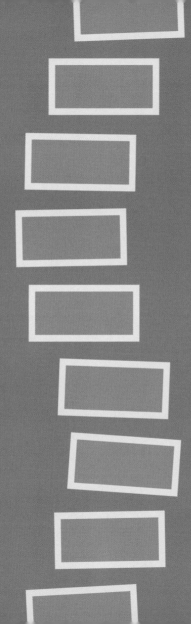

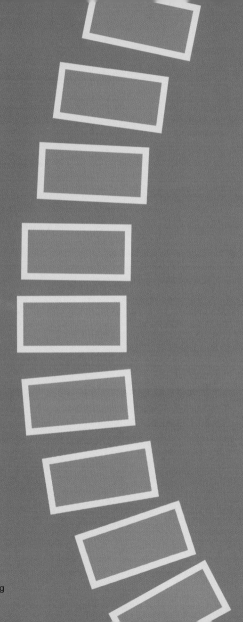

sitting

Sitting in a chair is not a position the human body was designed to do well. More natural positions to maintain an upright spine and head are squatting on your haunches, sei-za, the formal Japanese kneeling position, and the lotus position from yoga. However, both these positions require very high degrees of flexibility in the legs. Even though we may be able to learn to sit in these positions, we live in a culture that is not suited for floor-level living. We cannot change the customs of our culture, but we can make sure we don't carry poor postural habits once we are standing.

working surfaces

If the position of the head on the spine is to be maintained, it is important for work equipment, in particular the heights of keyboards and monitors, to be correct. The screen should be at eye level, so that there is no need to tilt the head back or forward to view it. Similarly if your work involves a lot of writing, drawing, or reading, it would be wise to invest in an inclinable worktop, such as a professional drawing table or a book rest.

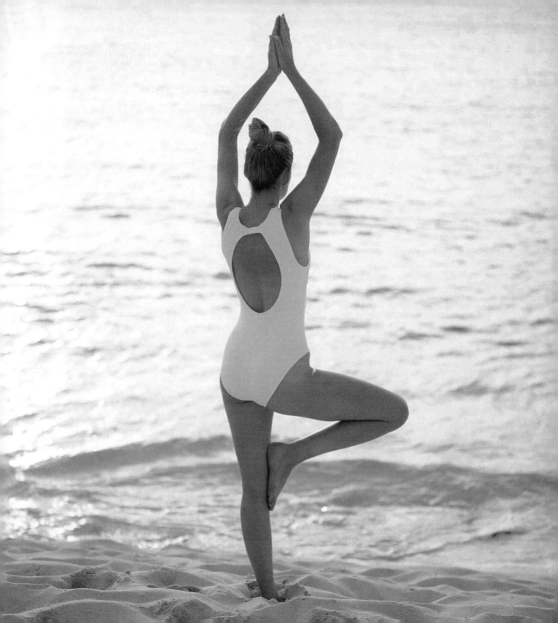

Simple exercises illustrating the principles of Alexander Technique

sitting

The usual way When we sit down, we usually start from the head. We jerk it back, then we stick out our backside, bending from the waist, and fall backwards. To slow the fall, we raise our heels off the floor and tighten our thigh muscles. This is a simple example of a "bad habit," which though not necessarily dangerous or wrong, is extremely wasteful in terms of energy.

The Alexander way When sitting or standing, the head and neck must be free of tension and in balance on top of the spine. Instead of falling down onto the chair with a thud, the idea is to use the alignment of the knee and hip joint to lower and raise yourself safely and with remarkably little effort. (AT applies the same principle to picking heavy objects from the ground, which is the cause of many a back injury.) The trick, though it's unlikely you'll be able to do it without some AT lessons, is to bend the hip (not the waist) and knees joints at exactly the same time. If you succeed, you should feel no tension in the thigh muscles, and your feet should stay firmly planted on the ground.

balance

A good way to test your alignment is to perform the tree, a yoga asana used to improve balance and concentration.

1   Stand with your feet together and arms by your sides. Seeking a fixed point ahead of you, focus your attention on it and do not allow your eyes and mind to wander.

2   Breathe in and place your right foot on the inside of your left leg, as high as is comfortable, with the knee pointing outward. Breathe out and move your hands overhead.

3   On the next out-breath, bring your hands into prayer position in front of your chest. Hold the pose for a minimum of five slow breaths.

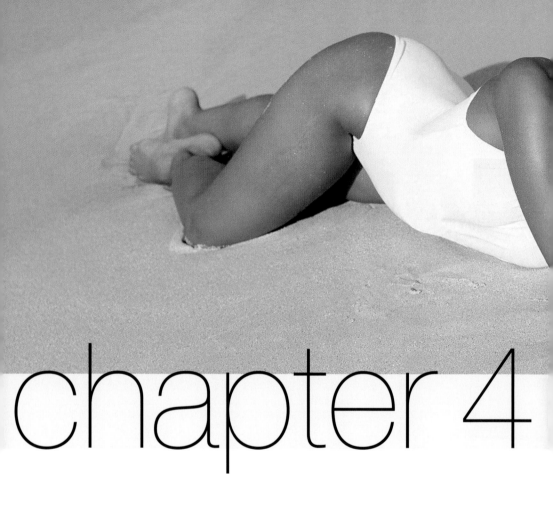

chapter 4

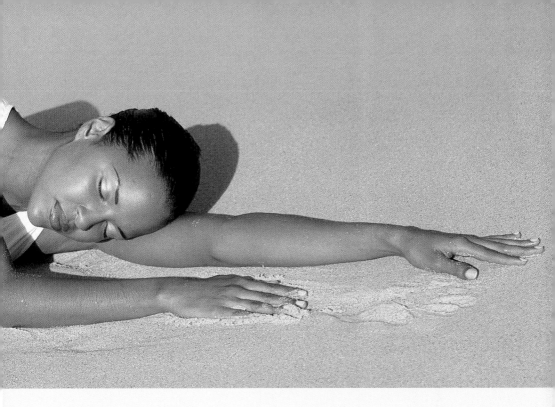

right action: flexibility

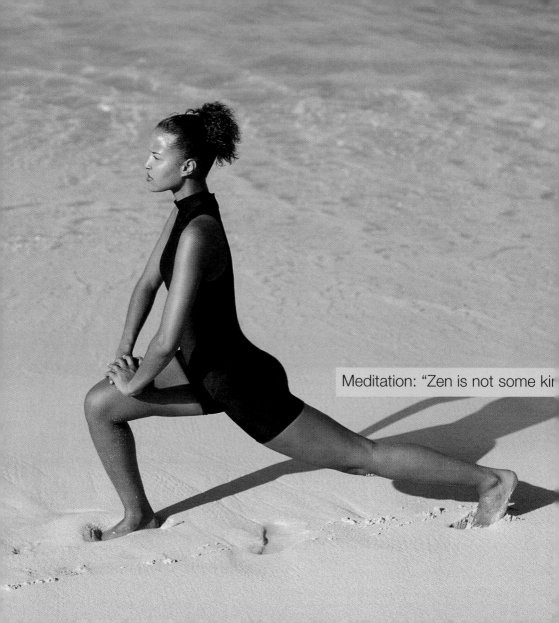

Meditation: "Zen is not some kir

excitement, but concentration on your usual everyday routine." —Shunryu Suzuki

In conventional, Western physical fitness culture, flexibility has been strength and endurance's poor relation. But to my mind, it is one of the foundations of both mental and physical fitness, and therefore of well-being. In physical terms, flexibility means the ability to move and change direction at a moment's notice with the minimum of disruption or risk of injury. On the mental level, flexibility is needed in your approach to work, relationships, and lifestyle, if you are to move smoothly through the stages of the human life cycle.

story

rag doll man

As it was a fine summer day, with no chance of rain, the man had decided that the time had come to change the broken tiles on the roof of his two-story suburban house. He had just carried his tools up to the roof and was stepping back onto the ladder to fetch the new tiles, when he lost his footing and fell toward the concrete path some 30 feet below. Luckily, his neighbor witnessed the accident. He immediately phoned the paramedics, certain that the fall onto the concrete had either killed his neighbor outright or left him badly injured.

The paramedics arrived within minutes, but the victim was not stretched out on the path where they expected to find him. He and his neighbor were in the kitchen having a cup of tea. He seemed shaken by the fall but generally unhurt. The paramedics, however, insisted that he go with them to the hospital for X-rays just in case he was not aware of his own injuries because he was in shock. The man smiled affably and let them take him to the hospital. A thorough examination revealed nothing more than a couple of cracked ribs and some extensive bruising. He was bandaged up and sent home.

The next day the local paper carried an article on its front page, under the headline "Miraculous escape of local resident," describing the circumstances of the accident. Embarrassed by what he saw as wholly undeserved attention, the man had given only the briefest of answers to the reporter's questions, agreeing that he had indeed been "incredibly lucky" to escape the fall without major injury. The reporter had had to make do with the sensationalistic account of the accident from the next door neighbor, who was clearly delighted to have become the center of attention. There was only one mention of what the man did for a living, which appeared at the very end of the article: "...he is a father of two, and is a yoga instructor."

The nest time I attended my weekly class at the Yoga Institute, the whole place was in uproar. A student of the institute had come across the item by chance, and now copies were circulating from class to class, much to the mortification of our teacher, who still failed to see what all the fuss was about. As he walked into the studio, he saw that he had twice the number of students he usually had. It was so crowded that we had to move to the Institute's largest studio.

Although everyone agreed that he was one of the Institute's most able teachers, his class was not the most popular with the students. He was a strict teacher who never pandered to his students' foibles nor tried to entertain them. On this occasion, he realized that he would not get any work out of his class if he did not say something about the accident, so in a complete break with his normal reserve about talking about himself, he told us the whole story.

There had been no time for conscious thought in the few seconds he had on the way down, he explained, but his body had taken over. Instead of tensing up for the impact, as a normal person would have done, thereby shattering every bone in his body, he went into savasana, the corpse pose, in which the body is completely relaxed. He hit the ground as limp as a rag doll, and the impact, instead of being absorbed by outstretched limbs, was distributed evenly over his entire body. Thus, he had survived the accident practically unscathed. He did not see anything extraordinary in his escape, and certainly did not consider it a "miracle," merely the practical application of the discipline he had spent many years perfecting. Quite to the contrary, it almost seemed that he would have been more surprised had he been injured by the fall.

Yoga

The word yoga is derived from the Sanskrit root yuj, which means to bind, join, attach, and yoke: to direct and concentrate one's attention on, to use and apply; a secondary meaning is "union" and "communion." According to the Indian academic Mahadev Desai, yoga represents, "The yoking of all powers of the body, mind, and soul to God... the disciplining of the intellect, the mind, the emotions... a poise of the soul which enables one to look at life in all its aspects evenly."

Although most Westerners think of yoga as an Asian exercise technique, it is in fact a religion. We do not recognize it as such because of the separation that exists in our own culture between body and spirit—a distinction that is quite alien to Asian thought. Like the t'ai chi ch'uan and chi kung (see pages 72–75) of China, yoga is based on an alternative view of human physiology that has a built-in spiritual dimension.

spiritual energy

India's traditional medicine, Ayurveda (science of life), has been in use on the subcontinent since about 2,500 BC. It has many elements that are reminiscent of the theories of yin and yang, chi, and the meridians that are found in traditional Chinese medicine.

In Ayurvedic belief, all living things are composed of the five elements—ether, air, fire, water, and earth—that are in constant flux. These can be simplified into the three dosha or vital energies: vata, pitta, and kapha. We humans are made up of combinations of the three vital energies, but one type is seen to predominate in each individual human being. The levels of the three dosha rise and fall in a daily cycle, in response to food intake, time of day, stress, and emotional state. Imbalances in the doshas disrupt the flow of prana (life energy), which can lead to mental and physical illness.

Prana, like chi, enters the body with air and food. It is distributed throughout the body by a system of 72,000 nadi, or energy channels. The central and most important channel of the subtle body passes through seven chakras (energy centers) that form a line from the base of the spine to the crown of the head and are connected to the main organs and glands. Focusing on the chakras during meditation and yoga regulates the flow of prana. This not only maintains health, but it also increases spiritual awareness. The Ayurvedic tradition believes that illness is caused by the build up of toxins within the body that upsets the balance of the patient's dosha. The emphasis in treatment is often on detoxification through herbal remedies, yoga, massage, and meditation.

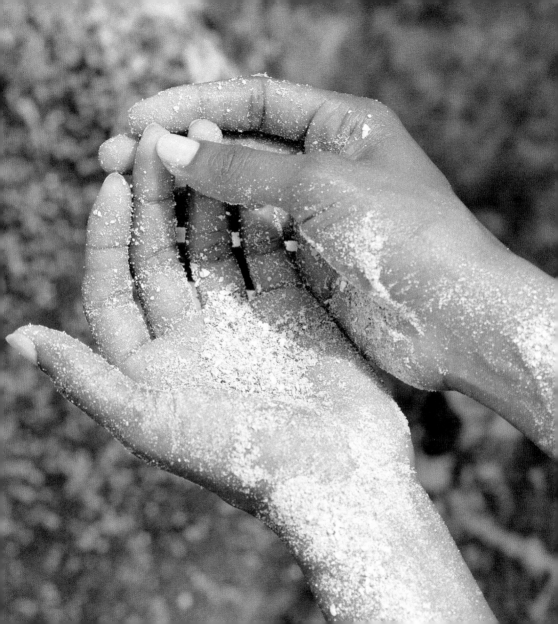

illness from within

An important consequence of the idea of prana as a spiritual energy, whose accumulation leads to enlightenment, is that an individual's mental and physical health (and his well-being), are equated with his spiritual development. If a person's dosha is unbalanced, and this has affected his prana, then he is not just physically ill but spiritually polluted as well. If this is translated into Western Christian terminology, we would have to say that a person who has fallen ill has incurred the wrath of God, and is being punished—an idea that has very little modern appeal, except to the most fundamentalist of Christian believers.

attacked from outside

Although in its own terms, it is a logical, coherent system, Ayurveda, like traditional Chinese medicine, represents a series of prescientific metaphors to explain the functions of the body, such as the circulation of the blood, respiration, and the nervous system. In its understanding of illness, unsurprisingly, it is ignorant of pathogens such as viruses and bacteria. The recent popularity of Ayurveda must be seen in the same light as the success of other non-Western therapies in employing the positive aspects of the mind-body link (see placebo effect, pages 88–89).

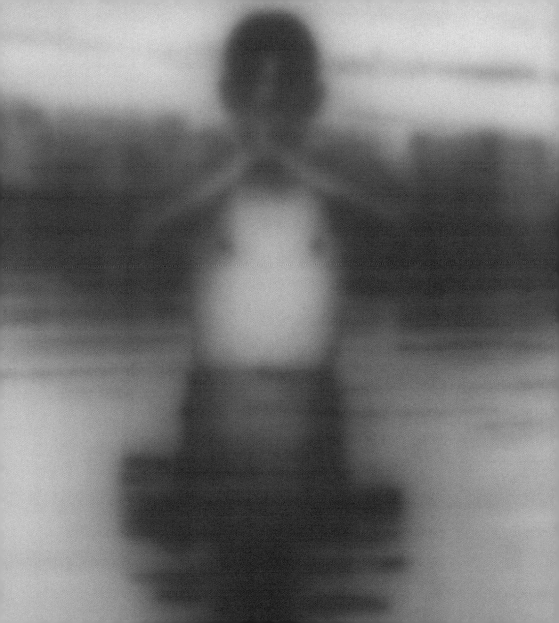

The yoga I studied was hatha yoga, which was taught not as a purely physical discipline but as the first stage of a spiritual pilgrimage toward enlightenment. For those who practice yoga regularly, they do not have to be great believers in the spiritual element of yoga to experience dramatic improvements in strength, flexibility, body shape, and self-image.

practicing yoga

During my stay in India, I had lost interest in the religious beliefs that underpin the practice of yoga. I continued to perform the asanas or poses, however, because their practice brought me a very concrete feeling of well-being that I wanted to explore further. But it was only several years later, after graduating from college, that I met someone with the same, almost intuitive, understanding of the power of flexibility training.

the desire to

In the early 1980s I joined the new YMCA in London, which in addition to the free-weights' room, had machine-weights, a swimming pool, basketball and squash courts, and several exercise studios with a full program devoted to the new aerobics.

I first met Sue in the coffee bar that overlooked the club's swimming pool. It was still early in the gym day—about 10 a.m.—but she had already finished, and was drinking her post-workout cup of tea. She was a regular every morning, and I often arrived about the time she was finishing her routine. Physically, there was nothing unusual about her. She was somewhere between pretty and plain, and someone less charitable would have said that she was slightly overweight. In every way she was an average woman of 28.

As we saw each other most days, we soon began to chat. It turned out that she had joined a few months before me. When we got to know each other a little better, she confided that she had reached a turning point in her life. Parting from the man she had lived with for eight years, she had also just sold her hairdressing business. She was not

stretch

sure where she wanted to go career-wise, but she knew it had to be something to do with physical fitness. She did not like the dance aerobics that were becoming popular at the time, because she felt uncoordinated and ungraceful, but she was taking a lot of different classes at the club and at a nearby dance center. She did reveal one ambition, however, which was to achieve the box splits—the full opening of the hip joint to the side.

Over the next few months our visits sometimes overlapped. Her morning routine consisted almost entirely of stretching exercises, several of which she had picked up from dance or aerobics classes, while others I recognized as modified yoga asanas. She performed this eclectic collection in her own way, adding and subtracting exercises, following some inner direction that brooked no outside criticism or advice. Although women are generally believed to be more flexible than men, I do not think that Sue, when she began stretching, had any significant advantage. She had no background in sport, exercise, or dance that would have given her a head start.

transformation

As I began to work full time, our meetings became less frequent, because our schedules no longer matched up. Finally, I went to work abroad. I returned a year and a half later, and renewed my membership. The day after rejoining, I came in at the time I knew Sue would be starting. I was not surprised to see her stretching at her usual place on the balcony above the main hall, but I was stunned when I actually joined her there and saw her face-to-face after an absence of eighteen months.

She was transformed. Somehow, she seemed not only to have stopped the ageing process, but to have actually reversed it. There were three things about her that I noticed at once:

- she had lost the excess body-fat that she had been carrying;
- her skin was more delicate and clearer than it had ever been—it had the almost translucent quality of baby skin;
- her posture was completely different. It was as if someone had dismantled her, stretched her out, and put her back together again.

She sat tall, head and back erect, but not in the forced manner of someone who is holding himself "at attention," but completely naturally. Had I known about Alexander Technique (see page 110), I would have guessed that she had studied it, but all she had done was follow her own instincts to exercise and stretch. She had achieved through exercise what men and women are willing to pay a fortune for in cosmetic surgery, and the completely natural result was better than the best surgeons could ever hope to equal.

As for the mental changes, they were almost as drastic. The hesitant person who had no clear idea of the direction her life was going to take and who lacked the self-confidence and assertiveness to make a decision was gone. She had been replaced by a smiling young woman, whose calmness and self-assurance drew people to her. I have always judged an activity by its results, and in this case, I had to admit that I was truly impressed. I was determined to discover what had wrought such a magical transformation.

the benefits of stretching

- increases vitality
- protects from injury
- increases flexibility
- strengthens the body and improves muscle tone
- re-aligns the body so that it functions effectively
- assists in the elimination of lactic acid in the muscles
that causes muscle cramps and post-training aches and pains
- regulates the internal organs, keeping all systems functioning efficiently
- slows the ageing process
- enhances concentration
- fights depression

intuitive stretchi

Sue was always the first to arrive in the morning. She had never set out to have pupils or teach; she did her routine every day at the same time. In my absence, she had acquired a group of admirers who came to train alongside her. Within a few months of my return, she would be teaching her own class at the dance center where she had studied, and her pupils would include ballet and jazz dancers, as well as other movement teachers. She had no pretensions about what she did, and she entitled the class "stretching." She could never be accused of being an intellectual in her training, nor of claiming any spiritual "insights." In all that she did, she was completely practical and pragmatic.

I made a point of joining Sue whenever I could and following her training routine. She would always start the same way, with standing leg stretches—the kind a ballet dancer performs on the bar—which she did on the balustrade of the balcony. She went on to forward bends that were more yoga based, but which she performed dynamically rather than statically. She swung back and forth as if hinged at the hips, and her hamstrings and lower back were loose enough that her torso hung vertically, without any rounding of the spine. I

ng

could see now why her posture was so good. She would then begin her floor work. After the seated hamstring stretches and shoulder stretches, came the hip stretches: the side and box splits. She was already pretty close to having a 90-degree opening of her hip joints, but she wanted to open them even further. From the box splits, she would roll forward onto her stomach. Her hips would be raised slightly off the mat, and this is the gap that she wanted to close. I would help her by pressing down on her legs from behind, gradually increasing the pressure until I was using almost all of my 175-pound weight to press her into the mat. Although she was much lighter, her full weight on my hips was sometimes excruciating, yet for reasons that we could not understand, we would joyfully continue with this torture.

The musculature of the legs is the strongest in the body, and the tendons holding the muscles to the bones, are some of the thickest. To open the hips fully was a slow and painful process. We often brought each other to the verge of tears, but we quickly realized these were not being prompted by the physical discomfort alone.

releasing
emotional pain

Unconscious, a human body can be manipulated into
any position. It is the tension in our muscles that holds us in
shape. Sue believed that this tension was emotional in origin—
a result of the mental stress that we had experienced during our
earlier lives that had somehow become locked into our bodies.
The pain we experienced was part physical and part emotional.
During a particularly hard session, we would often feel moved—
sometimes saddened, at others elated—as if we were reaching
down into ourselves and reliving deeply buried emotional states,
both happy and sad. She had come to this belief from her
own experiences of stretching, and not because she
had heard of the theories of physical therapists
such as Moshe Feldenkrais, Joseph Heller,
and Ida Rolf, who had come to very
similar conclusions.

rolfing

Working in Boulder, Colorado, during the 1960s and 1970s, Ida Rolf developed a theory of how emotional disturbance could affect the body, and created a system of massage, later known as "Rolfing," that would release it. It has long been known that the fibers that make up muscle tissue are separated into bundles by thin connective tissue known as fascia. Rolf proposed that when the body is subjected to physical or mental stress, the fascia lose their elasticity so that movement becomes increasingly restricted. This process is gradual; the person is unaware that it is taking place, and the body adapts to cope with the limitations that increase year by year. As the problem gets worse, however, breathing, posture, and movement all deteriorate, leading to declinng health and premature aging. In effect, what Sue and, to a lesser extent I, were doing in our experiments with stretching, was akin to "Rolfing" one another.

end note

My chronological age at time of writing is forty-three, but my actual age, in terms of appearance as well as my scores in standard tests for flexibility, aerobic fitness, and strength, is between five and ten years less. Of course, I cannot prove that I would not have stayed younger had I never stretched. There is no double-blind control trial that can be carried out on me to prove that I am not just genetically advantaged. And Sue? I see her infrequently, but each time, her youthfulness continues to astound me. She got married in her late thirties and moved away to live on the coast of England. At the age of forty, she had a son. Now, about to turn fifty, she has aged, of course, but not in the way that other women of her generation have. She retains the splendid posture and poise that she acquired twenty years ago. She continues to do her regular routine every morning, and teaches a stretching class to a new generation of pupils.

"Ah but I was so much older then;
I'm younger than that now."

—Bob Dylan

basic flexibility guidelines

Flexibility has long been relegated in Western sports culture to a secondary place, often added to workouts as an afterthought. Many people see flexibility as necessary only for specialized athletes, such as gymnasts, and for dancers. In all sports and exercise, however, good flexibility not only improves overall performance, it also protects the body from injury. It also has well-researched benefits for stress-related conditions. Flexibility training should be a daily activity, more like brushing one's teeth than going for a run or a workout. The benefits of stretching are cumulative, so a small amount—say 15 minutes—of daily stretching will be better than a weekly, hour-long stretching or yoga class.

clothing and equipment

- Loose, layered clothing is preferred in cold climates rather than the nude stretching one can do in the tropics. Make sure that the clothing you wear constricts none of the joints of your body.
- Practice on a padded stretching mat, as a towel or blanket will not provide enough protection for your skin as you stretch.

Stretching is one of the best preparations for the day, but early-morning stretchers should take care to warm the body up thoroughly before attempting the more difficult stretches on the following pages.

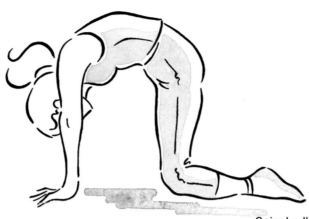

Spinal roll 1

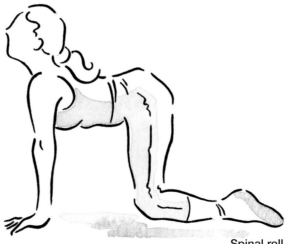

Spinal roll 2

basic flexibility workout

back

Spinal roll

1 Kneel on all fours, with your arms and thighs forming right angles with your torso. Starting from the base of the spine, round your back as much as possible and drop your head.

2 Starting from the base of your spine, slowly hollow your spine and raise your head. Repeat three times.

Spinal twist

1 Lie on your back with your arms straight out to the side.

2 Bend your legs and bring your knees to your chest. Keeping your shoulders on the floor, lower your knees to the right and turn your head to the left. Hold for at least 30 seconds. Repeat on the left side.

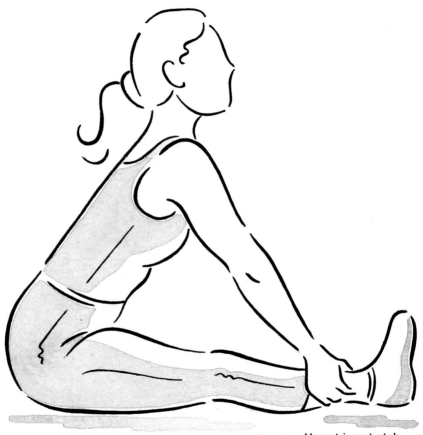

Hamstring stretch

basic flexibility workout

arms

Upper arm and shoulder stretch

1 Sit on the floor with your legs straight. Place your hands behind you, shoulder-width apart, fingers pointing away from your body.

2 Slide your body forward as far as it will go. Hold for 30 seconds.

Legs

Hamstring stretch

1 Sit with your legs outstretched, feet together. Keep your head and upper back erect.

2 Lean forward from the hips, and grab hold of your legs as far down as possible. Hold for at least 30 seconds.

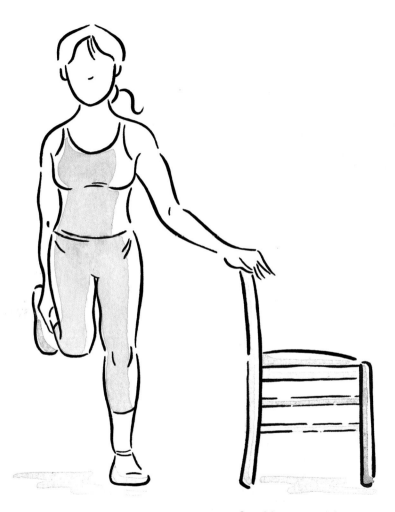

Quadriceps stretch

basic flexibility workout

Quadriceps stretch

1 Stand with your feet together.

2 Keeping your balance (hold onto a stationary object if necessary) bend your right knee and lift your right foot up behind you. Grab your foot with your right hand and pull it toward your body, making sure to keep your knees together and to keep your body upright. Hold for 30 seconds.

3 Repeat with the left leg.

Butterfly

1 Sit with your legs in front of you. Bring the soles of your feet together as close as possible to your body.

2 Keeping your head and body upright, put your hands on your thighs and push your legs down, trying to touch the floor with your knees. Hold for 30 seconds.

3 Hold your feet with your hands and lean forward, bending from the hips, keeping your head and back upright. Hold for 30 seconds.

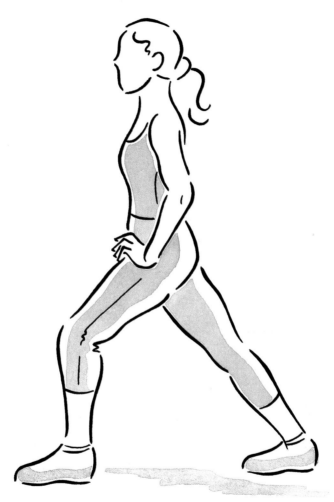

Lower leg stretch

basic
flexibility
workout

Box splits

1 Sit with your legs as far apart as possible, with your legs straight and flat on the floor. Hold for 30 seconds.

2 Keeping your head and back straight, place your hands in front of you on the floor and lean forward. Hold for 30 seconds.

Lower leg stretch

1 From a standing position, feet shoulder-width apart, take a large step forward with your right foot, hands on your hips. Keeping your feet flat on the floor, push forward with your hips to stretch the lower leg.

2 Step in with the back leg, and bend the back knee to stretch the Achilles tendon.

sun salutation sequence

1 Stand with your feet together, toes touching, heels an inch apart. Breathe in.

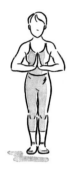

2 Breathe out and place your hands palms together in front of your chest in prayer position.

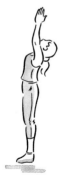

3 Breathe in and raise your arms above your head. Looking up at your hands, arch back as far as it is comfortable to go.

4 Exhale and bend forward with a straight back, bringing your hands to the floor on the outside of your feet. Bend your knees if necessary.

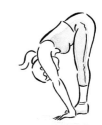

5 Bend your knees, exhale and take a large step back with your right leg. Extend your right foot back, and raise your arms above your head.

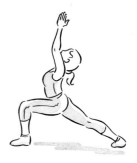

6 Lower your arms, put your hands on the floor, and bring your left foot back to join the right. Your body should now be in a push-up position, back flat, supported on hands and toes.

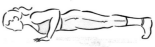

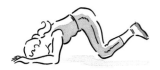

7 Exhale as you bring your torso up from the ground. Keeping your buttocks high, touch the floor with your forehead.

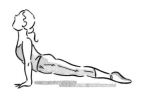

8 Inhale as you drop your hips and slide forward through your arms. Supporting your body with your hands, but without allowing your shoulders to rise to your ears, arch back as far as is comfortable. Keep your elbows bent.

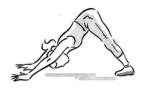

9 Breathe out, straighten your arms and legs and raise your buttocks as high as they will go without lifting your feet from the floor. Look back to your feet.

10 Inhale as you bring your right foot forward between your hands. Raise your arms above your head.

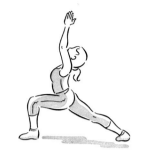

11 Lower your arms, exhale, and bring your left foot next to your right foot. Straighten your knees as much as possible.

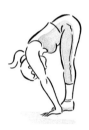

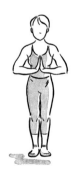

12 Breathe in and raise up with a flat back, bring your arms above your head, and arch back as far as is comfortable. Then exhale and lower your arms to the prayer position.

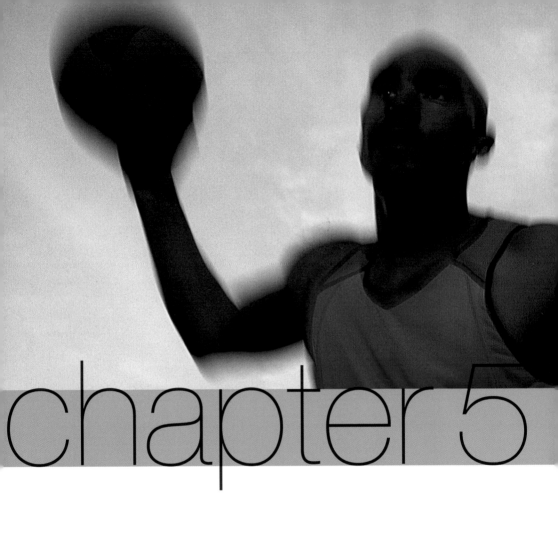

chapter5

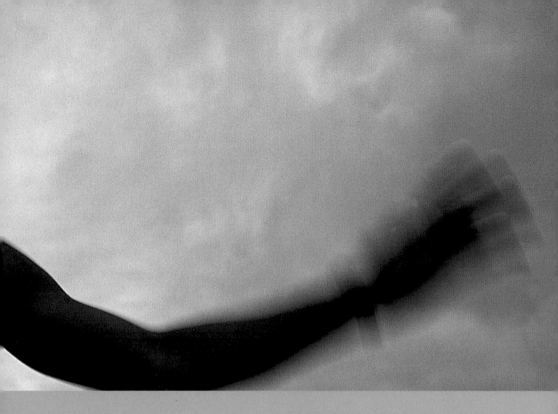

right speech: stamina

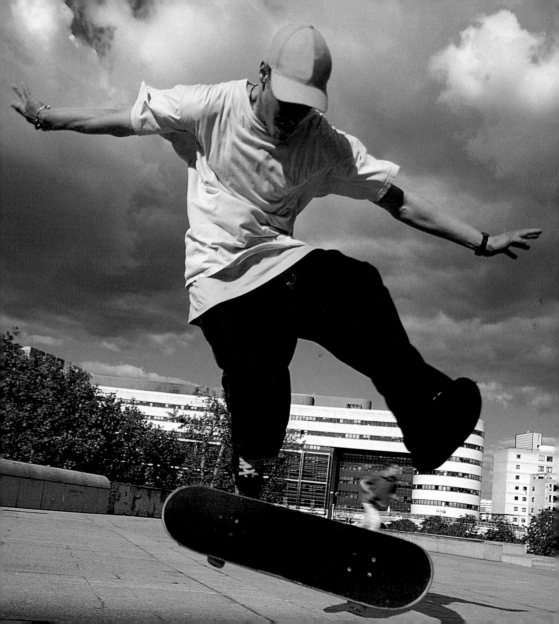

Meditation: "You will go most safely in the middle way."—Ovid

Endurance, or aerobic fitness is one of the three vital ingredients of physical well-being. In addition to the direct protection it affords to the heart and arterial system, aerobic health has a role to play in slowing the ageing process, controlling stress and body weight, and maintaining general health. Because of the conveniences of modern life, however, the types of activity that sustains and develops heart-lung fitness, such as walking and manual labor, have largely disappeared. We now have to create opportunities to train for endurance, but these are fraught with pitfalls, and sometimes, in our pursuit of health and fitness, we achieve the exact opposite. As in all of life's activities, let balance and moderation be your guides.

iron in the soul

The supporters of the Kyoto Triathlon Club packed into the club's microbus and several cars for the early morning drive to Lake Biwa for the annual Biwa Ironman Triathlon race. It was mid-August, the hottest time of year in Japan, with temperatures in the 90s and humidity close to 90 percent. The kind of heat that leaves you dripping with sweat even when standing still. The day dawned fine, without a cloud in the sky, and even at 7 A.M. as we drove off, the heat haze shimmered just over the highway.

Seven of the club's members were competing in the race that year: four men and three women, one of whom, Ayako-chan, a twenty-one-year-old aspiring Japanese champion, was hoping to finish among the first ten women. A regular competitor, she had been training hard for the event. At the other end of the fitness scale was Kimura-san, my calligraphy teacher, who had joined the club a year earlier, and was participating in her very first triathlon. To look at her, Kimura-san was the last person you would take to be a triathlete. She was a woman in her mid-30s, whose level of fitness left something to be desired. Her training had been erratic, and although the general opinion in the club was that she was not fit enough to complete the race, she was determined to participate. Not even her partner, who was also taking part in the race, had managed to talk her out of it.

I had arrived in Kyoto too late to sign up for the race, but I was secretly relieved. The Ironman is the toughest event in the triathlon calendar, with event distances of around one and a half miles for the swim, eighty-eight miles for the cycle ride, followed by a full marathon (twenty-six miles). However, as a regular on the club's weekly cycle sessions these past three months, I was more than happy to tag along to support the team.

Although I had seen many races on television, this was the first time I would be attending one in person. Lake Biwa is a splendid backdrop for this yearly event. The largest lake on the main Japanese island of Honshu, Biwa is ringed by mountains, and its shoreline is dotted with the ruins of castles that testify to the area's crucial importance during Japan's medieval period. The cycling and running courses around the lake are predominantly flat. Although this makes Biwa less challenging than some Ironman courses, the risk of dehydration from the intense summer heat is a very real threat to the competitors. Few spectators had turned out to see the race live. Most, I imagined, would be friends and family of the competitors. What the crowd lacked in numbers, however, was more than made up by the buzz of the media entourage, officials, and major corporate sponsors that every major international sporting event now attracts.

Triathlon racing is a relatively recent introduction to Japan, but its concentration on endurance makes it particularly attractive to Japanese competitors. While the Australian, American, and European stars of the Ironman circuit were present, the bulk of the amateur participants were Japanese.

The competitors had set off even earlier, and had already changed into their wet suits when we reached the spot at the lakeside where the swimming part of the event was to be held. There were several hundred competitors—all selected by lottery, such is necessary nowadays because so many people want to participate in even these most grueling of events. The swimmers, in bathing caps and goggles, their numbers magic-markered on their upper arms for easy identification, looked like a flock of strange, flightless, albino seabirds as they crowded into the water, jostling for the best position close to the start line.

the swim

The starting gun set off a stampede of bodies into the water. The professional racers, Ayako-chan among them, quickly split off from the mass of amateurs. The course went straight out to a buoy, and then along the shoreline before turning back to shore to the landing point where the bikes were ready for the second stage of the race.

The gleaming, brightly colored triathlon bikes, parked in bike racks in rows, waited for the competitors. While the stragglers were still barely halfway through the swim, the leaders were already emerging from the water, throwing aside bathing caps and goggles with little regard where they might fall. Drying in the sun, they struggled into shoes and cycling helmets before jumping onto their machines.

We watched and cheered our team members as they emerged from the water. Ayako-chan, much to our delight, was among the first ten women. She was so concentrated on the race that she did not to see us. Despite our fears, Kimura-san, whom we expected to come close to the end, emerged in the middle of the pack. She acknowledged our cheers, and then looked momentarily confused. She could not find her bike. We signaled frantically, directing her to her bike, which was kept in competitor number order.

the cycle ride

Once all the team members had ridden off, we ourselves departed. In good Japanese fashion, the club's president had decided that we should split up into groups to cheer on the team at strategic points around the 88-mile circuit. With two companions for company, I was stationed 25 miles from the start, so I saw all the team pass by.

Although it was still barely 10 A.M., the sun was beginning to heat up in earnest. We crouched in the shade of the car, standing up when we saw the leaders coming along the road toward us. As the terrain was flat, we could see them coming from several miles away. They seemed to take an age to reach us, but when they did, they flashed past, oblivious to our cries of encouragement. The faster amateurs were half an hour behind them. Ayako-chan came first among the club's team, a look of grim determination on her face, but she had already fallen behind the ten leading women. The plucky Kimura-san, as we feared, brought up the rear of the team, and was falling back in the order of the race.

All around the course, the toll of casualties was beginning to mount because of equipment failures and injuries. Fortunately, none of our team suffered anything more serious than punctures of their racing bikes' ultra-thin tires. We assembled again at the finishing line for the cycling stage to watch the start of the final running stage.

The lead riders swept into view. The American world champion was again first, followed by an Australian and several Japanese challengers. After an eighty-eight-mile ride, you might have expected them to pause, if only to acknowledge the cheers of the spectators, but the professionals were so intent on their times that they leapt off their bikes, swapped helmets and cycling shoes for running shoes and set off once more.

Ayako-chan had dropped even further back from the leading group of women, and came in somewhere between thirtieth and fortieth. We did not see Kimura-san arrive, because she had fallen so far behind the leaders that we had to leave to take our positions on the running course by the time she embarked on the last stage: the marathon.

The marathon derives its name from the heroic twenty-six-mile run of a soldier from the battlefield of Marathon to his home city of Athens, with news of the Greek victory against a vastly superior Persian force. In a telling conclusion to the the world's first ever marathon, the messenger died of exhaustion after relaying the news.

the marathon

Endurance events, such as the marathon and triathlon, are the ultimate tests of physical and mental fitness. Training for these events requires boundless stores of personal motivation to overcome the physical difficulties, as well as the mind-numbing boredom of the miles you have to cover on a daily basis in all weather. Unlike the Greek hero, today's competitors undergo the extremes of boredom, exhaustion, and dehydration, not to announce some portentous event, but, strangely, for the sheer pleasure of taking part.

Although the endurance racer's effort is admirable, it is self-destructive, and it will ultimately impact negatively on his or her well-being. The human body, although it is incredibly resilient, is not designed to take the kind of punishment that the long-distance events impose. Even in exceptionally genetically gifted individuals—the Olympic champions—the muscles strain, the ligaments and tendons tear, joints are ground down, and even the heart, which needs moderate, regular aerobic exercise, is often damaged and malfunctioning by the time the elite competitive athlete has reached middle age.

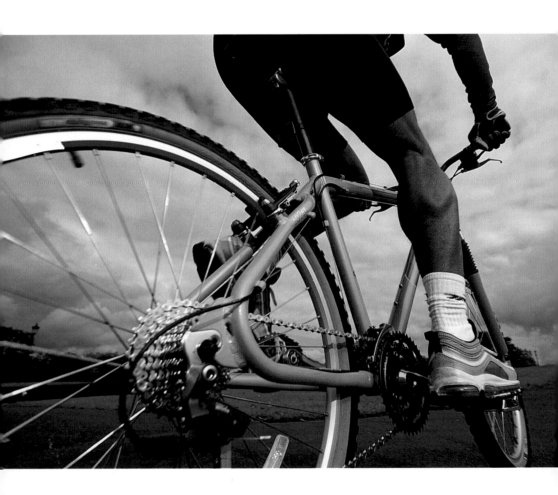

The psychological reward of winning, or "being the best," is not the only factor at play for the long-distance racer. It is now known that prolonged, intensive exercise, like running or cycling, will trigger the release of endorphins—the body's own natural opiates and the brain's very own pleasure-inducing and pain-relieving chemicals. In a very real sense, the endurance athlete can become addicted to his or her event. From the perspective of well-being, the endurance racer has lost the all-important balance that is needed in physical training. From the perspective of Zen, the strong likelihood that addiction is present renders the pursuit psychologically counterproductive. I am not, however, suggesting that no one should ever go for a run. Far from it, running is one of the most efficient ways I know of developing aerobic fitness. It requires little outlay in terms of expenditure, except for a good pair of shoes (see below), and it can be done in any location and at any time.

a balanced perspective

kamikaze spirit

Back on the shores of Lake Biwa, at the finishing line for the marathon stage of the Ironman triathlon, Ayako-chan crossed the line well behind the leading women, arriving sixty-seventh. As I ran up to congratulate her on finishing the race, she fell into my arms and burst into tears. To my amazement, she was inconsolable. She had just completed the full Ironman distance in under four hours, an amazing feat, but in her own terms she had failed utterly. The simple fact was that although young, and at the peak of her physical fitness, she had pushed herself too far. She had taken part in another race only two weeks before, not giving herself enough time to recover, and she had overtrained in the interval between the races.

Other team members finished one by one. Although they finished in times ranging between three-and-a-half and five hours, in contrast to Ayako-chan, they were delighted to have managed to finish the race, for most of them their first Ironman distance. We wrapped them in the sponsor's space-age metallic blankets, and led them to the competitors' rest area, where we had laid out a finishers' picnic.

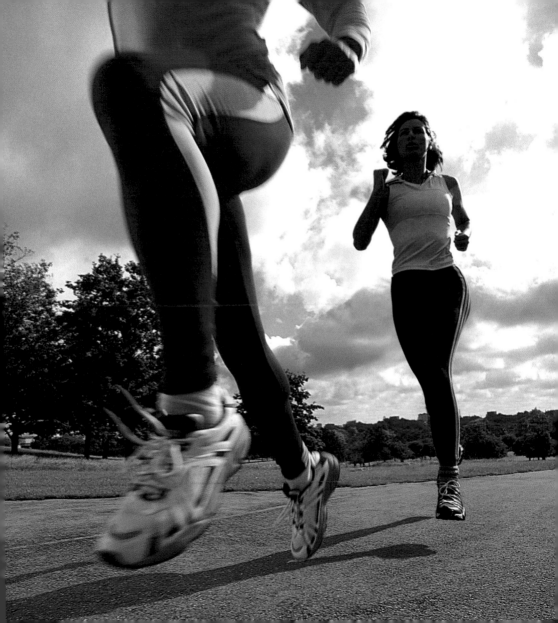

crossing the line

The day was well advanced as the last few runners crossed the line, but there were still a few competitors left unaccounted for, one of them, our very own Kimura-san. The large digital clock over the finishing line was counting up the seconds, minutes, and hours to twelve hours—the maximum time allowed to complete the race. Kimura-san had about two-and-a-half hours left before she would be disqualified.

For twenty minutes, there was no news of her, as the stewards contacted the way-stations along the route to try and discover her exact whereabouts. Unfortunately, by this time, most of the stations had packed up for the day, their job done, and their officials were on their way back to the finishing line. The organizers were just as much in the dark as we were. The only other missing competitor, a man in his 60s, limped across the finishing line to the cheers of the small crowd of spectators and officials. We began to speculate on possible scenarios. Had she given up? Was she lying injured in a ditch by the side of the road somewhere? Finally the press came to the rescue by redirecting its helicopter to survey the course.

Fifteen minutes later, the following announcement was made over the PA, "Competitor 2,032, Kimura-san of the Kyoto Triathlon Club, is 10 km away from the finishing line."
She had a little over two hours to finish. Plenty of time for someone to run three miles three

times over, under normal circumstances, but Kimura-san had just swum, cycled, and now run two-thirds of a marathon. A team member produced a portable radio, and picked up a local station. They were relaying special bulletins from the finishing line on Kimura-san's progress at regular intervals. The reporter told his listeners that although she was close to exhaustion, she was determined to finish the race. Soon he was announcing that she had slowed to a walk. For the following hour-and-a-half, we had nothing to do but wait, watching the time trickle away on the clock.

At last the news we were waiting for came. Kimura-san was less than a kilometer away. Seeing the finishing line in the distance, she picked up speed in a strange looking forward stagger. A doctor was running ahead of her, with two nurses alongside, spraying her legs with anaesthetizing cold spray. With fifteen minutes to spare, and a cheer much louder than the one that had greeted the race's winner, Kimura-san crossed the line and collapsed into her boyfriend's arms. She had gone a disturbing shade of gray and had to be carried to the rest area, but she had triumphed over the race, and over her own body's weakness.

gambare

The Japanese have a great admiration for people who push themselves beyond their physical limits. They even have a word, gambare ("try harder"), which describes this kind of spirit. Kimura-san had demonstrated a full measure of gambare in completing the Ironman, but, sadly, it was at a very high cost to herself. She was so exhausted that it took her several weeks to recover fully from the race. She had injured her knees and ankle joints, and did not return to the club for the rest of the time I trained with the Kyoto Triathlon Club.

Kimura-san had proved that the mind can triumph over matter for a limited time. Matter, however, always gets its own back in the end, and for a much longer period.

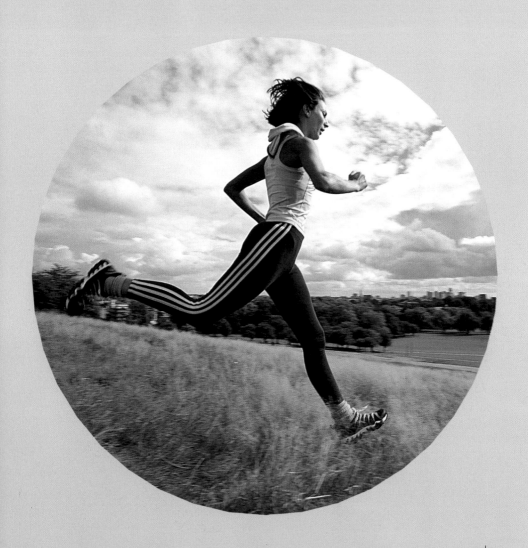

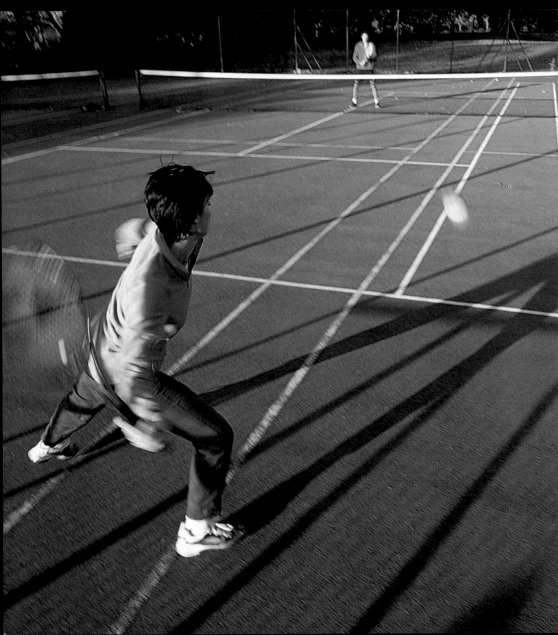

endurance training guidelines

The rule to follow in training for endurance or aerobic (heart-lung) training is to follow a program of regular, moderate exercise. Although the basic advice to train aerobically for twenty minutes three times a week still holds, health authorities in the developed world also recommend that people accumulate shorter periods of aerobic activity throughout the day. In addition to the three weekly runs or sessions on an aerobic simulator, you should, for example, take part in sports, cycle, run, or roller-blade instead of driving; walk upstairs instead of taking the elevator; and take up active hobbies, such as gardening.

Those people who wish to train their heart and lungs as efficiently as possible, will need to know their Aerobic Training Zone (ATZ) and be able to take their heart rate (HR) quickly. (See below for a simple method of calculating your HR during exercise.) An alternative is to purchase a pulse monitor, which consists of a chest-strap and a wrist unit, for a constant readout of your pulse. Most models will warn you as soon as you have left your AZT.

to work out your ATZ

1 Subtract your age from 220 to derive your maximum HR per minute, which you should not exceed in training.
e.g. for a person 30 years of age: 220 – 30 = 190 bpm (beats per minute).
2 Your ATZ, the range of HR within which you will obtain aerobic benefit, is 55–80 percent of your maximum heart rate.
e.g. for a person 30 years of age: 190 x 0.55 = 104; 190 x 0.8 = 152: ATZ = 104-152 bpm

taking your pulse during exercise

Press the index and middle fingers on the underside of your forearm, about two inches from your wrist, in the depression between the two forearm bones. Do not use your thumb to take the pulse as it has a strong pulse of its own and may give you a confusing reading. Count the number of heartbeats in ten seconds and multiply the result by six to obtain your heart rate per minute.

aerobic exercise and weight loss

If you are interested in aerobic training as a form of weight control, you are recommended a long, low-intensity workout at the lower end of your ATZ. A typical example would be a forty-five-minute to a one-hour walk or cycle, when you maintain your HR at around 55 percent of the maximum.

Aerobic Training Zone (ATZ)

running

aerobic training

Aerobic training can be very stressful physically, especially for beginners. It is essential to take the following points into consideration.

- Warm-up thoroughly (see page 95 for general warm-up guidelines and pages 158–165 for stretching), especially the joints and muscles most affected by the exercise chosen: hips, knees, and ankle joints for running; shoulders, elbows, and wrists for rowing.
- Wear appropriate clothing and equipment for the conditions. For running, it is essential to buy a running shoe with a cushioned sole to reduce the impact on the leg joints if running on a hard surface such as a road or sidewalk. Shoes designed for other activities, such as basketball and tennis shoes, are not suitable for running. They do not provide enough cushioning, and the more rigid design of the upper part of the shoe will impede a proper running action.

running technique

While all forms of aerobic exercise require good technique, poor technique in running is the cause of the majority of endurance training injuries. Typically a runner strikes the ground with the outside of his heel, which is the most heavily padded part of the shoe, the foot rolls through and the toes leave the ground for the next step. Some runners have a tendency to hit the ground flat-footed or on the inside of the heel, and both of these differences may require special footwear so as not to lead to injury.

As you run, your upper body should be relaxed, with your arms flowing easily in time with your stride. Make sure you do not tense your chest and shoulders, as this will adversely affect your breathing. Another point to look out for is the arm swing, which can be unbalanced and throw your running pattern off by tilting your torso to one side.

If you suffer from injuries or weaknesses in the leg joints or lower back, or are prone to shinsplints (painful inflammation of the lower leg) even in appropriate running shoes, then you should discontinue running and opt instead for an alternative form of aerobic exercise.

power walking

Providing the same benefits as running, power walking requires that you monitor your HR constantly to make sure you are walking fast enough to keep within your ATZ.

swimming

A very good alternative for someone with leg joint or lower back injuries, or a propensity for shinsplints. Swimming is the ultimate low-impact activity. However, this does not mean that it is injury free. There can be strain on the shoulder joints, and care should be taken to warm up thoroughly, especially before doing demanding strokes such as the backstroke and the butterfly.

cycling and in-line skating

Both are good alternatives to running, as long as you can maintain a steady pace for a sufficient period. Cyclists and skaters are more likely to suffer traumatic injuries from accidents and falls, and should always wear protective gear. Commuter cyclists and skaters, while they are improving their general fitness may not be improving their heart-lung fitness if their journeys are too short or involve too many stops and starts.

alternatives to running

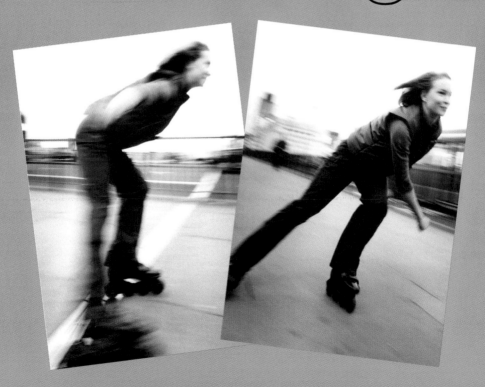

aerobic simulators

For many of us who do not have either the time or a suitable environment for an outdoor aerobic activity, the indoor aerobic simulator—stationary bikes, stairmaster, rowing machine, and running machine—are often the only available options. Although there is some slight variation in energy expenditure between machine types, especially when you begin training on an unfamiliar machine, this is not significant in the long run. Research has shown that the degree of familiarity with a piece of aerobic equipment will determine how many calories you use up during a training session: the less familiar you are with the equipment, the more calories you burn. A good practice is to vary the type of equipment you use on each training session.

In the past five years, manufacturers have tried to come up with several new formats for aerobic simulators. The most successful of these from the training point of view are the no-impact air walker and the elliptical trainer.

The following table gives you the types of equipment to avoid if you are susceptible to certain injuries.

Equipment	Avoid with injuries of:
Rowing machines	Back or neck
Stationary bikes	Knees
Running machines	Knees, ankles, shinsplints
Stairmaster	Knees, ankles

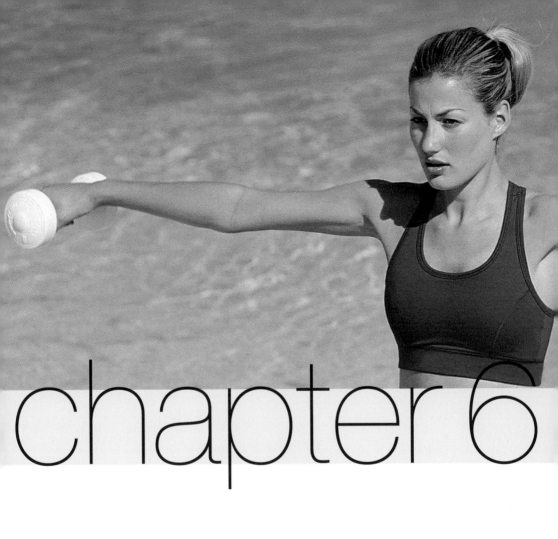

chapter 6

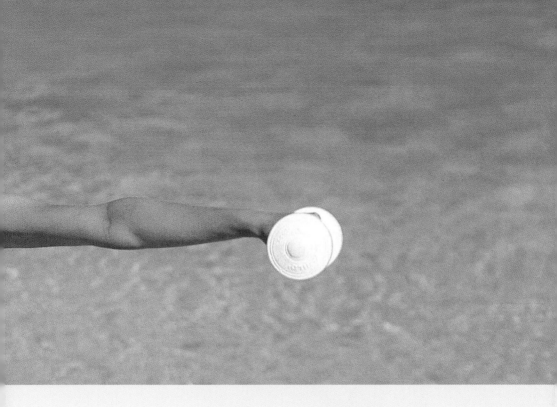

right effort: strength

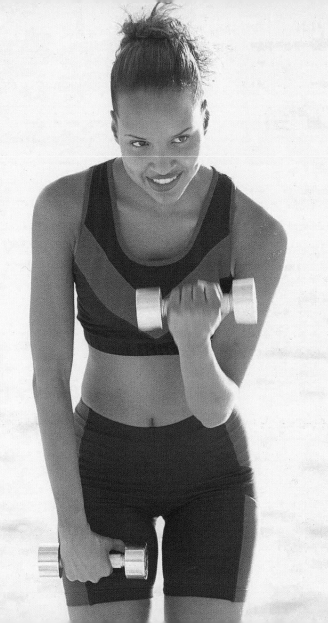

The final aspect of physical well-being is strength. Without a strong musculature, posture collapses, because the body lacks the power to stabilize the joints. Strength training—with one's own body weight, machine-weights, or free-weights—is the single most powerful technique available to transform your fitness and appearance. However, despite its popularity, it is one of the least understood and most poorly taught forms of exercise.

In order to get the most of any strength-building exercise, you have to know what muscles you are targeting, and how these operate the joints involved in the movement. The bench press, for example, is a classic free-weight exercise to train the chest. Its aim is to increase the strength and size of the two large, fan-shaped pectoralis major muscles that cover the upper part of the rib cage. The narrow part of the fan attaches on the clavicle bone of the shoulder and the broad end attaches along the length of the sternum and the ribs. The role of the pectoralis muscles is the horizontal adduction of the shoulder joint, or in layman's terms, moving the arms across the front of the body. Several secondary muscles, notably the triceps brachii (the muscles at the rear of the arms that straighten the arms from the elbows) are also brought into play.

Once function is understood, it is only a question of applying the proper

form and

function

"form" to the exercise. In the case of the bench press, the feet are flat on the floor, knees square, back flat on the bench, head supported. The barbell is lifted off the supports with a wider-than-shoulder-width grip, and brought to a position directly over the chest. Keeping the movement smooth and the speed constant, the bar is lowered to the chest so that it lightly touches the ribcage at the height of the nipples, to ensure that the maximum range of movement of the shoulder joints is used.

The second fundamental principle of strength training is that a muscle will only gain strength within the range of movement it is trained in. This means that if you habitually stop the pressing movement three inches above your chest, you will have developed the ability to lift more weight to that point. Should you then let the bar fall all the way down to your chest, in all likelihood, you will be unable to lift the bar off your chest.

"A fool can always
to admire him."

at a gym near you

The man on the bench press is straining under a weight that far exceeds his capacity to lift it. Encouraged by his comrades, however, he squares up under the barbell, and raises his hips off the bench, arching his lower back, so that it is his body that rises to meet the weight rather than the barbell that moves down smoothly to contact with his chest. He executes this movement four times, levering himself off the floor with his legs, each time going a little higher, and placing a greater strain on his lumbar vertebrae. His face contorted by one final supreme effort, he manages to heave the bar back onto the metal rack of the bench. He jumps up in triumph to the acclamation of his training buddies. The barbell has not moved more than three inches during each repetition of the exercise.

find a greater fool

—Nicolas Boileau

the cheat

From the brief description of form and function, it is clear that the man on the bench press is breaking every rule of proper weight training. He is actually using a recognized technique called "cheating," in which form is sacrificed to lift more weight. Although it is considered dangerous, cheating has a small part to play in advanced training for the professional bodybuilder or strength athlete, but it never replaces proper form as it has done so clearly here.

At some point in his training career, our "cheat" has decided that lifting the maximum amount of weight in certain exercises was more important than anything else he wanted to achieve.

This scene will be familiar to anyone who frequents a gym in the United States or Europe. On this occasion, however, I am in a municipal gym in Tokyo, proving conclusively that stupidity, when it comes to exercise, is not a monopoly of those raised within Western exercise culture. This man, and the many like him all over the world, has been weight training for approximately a decade. Somehow, he has missed the point of the activity.

A closer examination of his physique reveals that he is suffering from various afflictions common to cheats the world over: "chicken-leg syndrome"—in which the upper body is much more developed than the lower body, giving him an unbalanced appearance reminiscent of the anatomy of a chicken. He also has extremely rounded shoulders caused by the shortening of the chest muscles that pull the shoulders and head forward.

injury

As is usual in a gym—a social venue with its own customs and strict code of etiquette—the group at the bench press takes turns to do their sets. The others, I note, although their form is far from ideal, do not cheat to the same extent. The cheat's turn comes around once more. With great ceremony, he sits down on the bench for his next set. He squares up under the bar once more, and begins to arch his back off the bench while lifting the bar off the wrack. We hear a very distinct and surprisingly loud "Snap!" The cheat crumples up under the bar, which he somehow manages to hold aloft at arms' length. As in an animated cartoon, time seems to stop and the action seems to freeze, with the barbell hanging in mid-air like the 10-ton weight waiting to drop out of the sky on the unsuspecting victim. Fortunately, one of the spotters has the presence of mind to grab the barbell and yank it back onto the supports, thus preventing it from falling onto the cheat and adding to his injuries. The man rolls off the bench and lets out a single agonized yell.

Weight training is without a doubt the most powerful technique at our disposal to change both our general physical fitness and our appearance. In the cheat's case, he used it to gradually weaken his body, until in one catastrophic failure, it gave out on him. As we waited for the paramedics, I eavesdropped on his training-partners' conversation. "It was a piece of bad luck," one of them says, and the others nod in sage agreement. There will be no lesson learned here today, nor at the sites of thousands of similar injuries in gyms the world over. When the cheat is able to begin training again, I am certain he will not change his technique, because to do so would mean reducing the weight he is lifting by half.

loss of reality

The kind of dramatic injury I described on the previous pages is thankfully quite rare. But anyone who goes to a gym for any length of time will begin to experience minor ailments of the mind and body as a direct consequence of training. One particular weight trainer, Michael, constantly suffered with pain in the neck, shoulder, or back. As soon as one injury improved, it seemed, another would flare up, and his training was constantly interrupted. His recourse was to visit physiotherapists, osteopaths, and massage therapists for treatments. Although they could free him temporarily from the pain and release the stiffness that locked his muscles in place, within days, sometimes hours, both the aches and stiffness would return.

An osteopath finally told him to stop weight training altogether, but Michael's self-image was too bound up in his training, and despite the constant pain, he felt unable to stop. The cause of his injuries was not poor technique, and when he was able to train, he got extremely good results, but somehow his body was working against him.

As he trained, tension originating in his daily life seemed to become locked into certain parts of his body. This had two effects: instead of supporting the joints of his spine and shoulders, his musculature was pulling them out of shape. The second was that the constant muscular tension was constricting the blood vessels in the affected areas. This not only caused the muscles to work less efficiently, but it also prevented the removal of toxins, reduced the oxygen supply, and slowed down the healing process.

As with the "cheat," an unbreakable link had been forged in Michael's mind between his physical appearance and strength and his worth as a individual, and it would take more than pain, or even an accident, however serious, to sever that association.

Obsessive strength training belongs in that class of addictions to activities that are usually considered beneficial. Its physical consequences are the kind of injuries described above, but there is also a well documented "overtraining syndrome," with symptoms including moodiness, depression, insomnia, and loss of appetite.

abuse

When I had graduated university, I joined a bodybuilders' gym with Richard, a friend who had graduated a year ahead of me. Richard, a serious college swimmer, had been weight training for a year when I joined him. His body already showed some encouraging results. He had gained about ten pounds overall. His gains, however, disappointed him when he compared himself to the other men in the gym. I pointed out that they had been training for years, but he responded that he knew about a short-cut he could take. What he meant, naturally, was going on an illegal course of anabolic steroids that would further stimulate muscular growth by flooding his body with the male hormone testoterone. He assured me that he would do it just to "catch up" and encouraged me to do the same.

He chose the steroid Dekaduroboline (Nandralone), which is much in the news at present because it is commonly abused by track and field athletes. Coupled with huge increases in food intake, and intensive training, anabolic steroids allowed him to achieve a 10 to 15 percent increase in body weight. I was not surprised to hear that he later went back on his assurance that he would do only one course of steroids. He had become psychologically dependent not on the drug itself, which has no addictive properties, but on the gains in size and strength they gave him. Within a few years, he was competing and winning national bodybuilding competitions.

obsession

Although ultimately I did not share his ambitions, and we went our separate ways, for several months, I was also momentarily dazzled by the pursuit of size and strength. I was much too cautious to risk taking anabolic steroids, whose listed side-effects include baldness, acne, high blood pressure, and liver and kidney failure. I preferred to stick to the conventional route of intensive training, the most important part of which is a massive increase in calorie intake to allow the body to grow.

Rather than a free-for-all, with unlimited quantities of treats, such as cakes, cookies, fried food, and chocolates, however, my diet was as highly regulated as any weight-watcher's program. The bulk of my extra calorie intake was made up of carbohydrates and proteins. Two to three grams of protein per two and a quarter pounds of body weight, and one pound of extra carbohydrates for energy.

78 kg x 2 = 156g of protein/4 calories gram = 644 calories

500 g of carbohydrates/4 calories gram = 2,000 calories

644 + 2,000 + 1,850 BMR = 4,594 calories/day

In just four months of training, I had gained a respectable seventeen and a half pounds, with only a moderate increase in body fat percentage, and my body fat had remained well within the permissible 20 percent. To maintain the gains, however, I had to keep eating the extra calories, made up of lean sources of proteins (chicken breast, tuna, and egg whites) and large quantities of complex carbohydrates (pasta, bread, rice, and potatoes) without the benefit of the flavoring provided by fats and refined sugars.

It was like being an anorexic in reverse—overeating obsessively instead of starving obsessively. I wondered if anorexia and bodybuilding were not the two extremes of the same spectrum.

- Anorexics no longer wish to exist and will allow themselves to waste away to nothing.
- Bodybuilders, at the other extreme, want to become larger and larger, occupying more space in the world, as if greater size literally meant a greater access to life.

To make sure that I got the necessary calories and protein, I had to make a note of everything I ate. In the end, I was beginning to find it almost impossible to keep eating enough. I had reached a crossroads in my fitness career. One path was to follow Richard, go on a course of steroids and train for competition, the other would take me away from him in an entirely new direction.

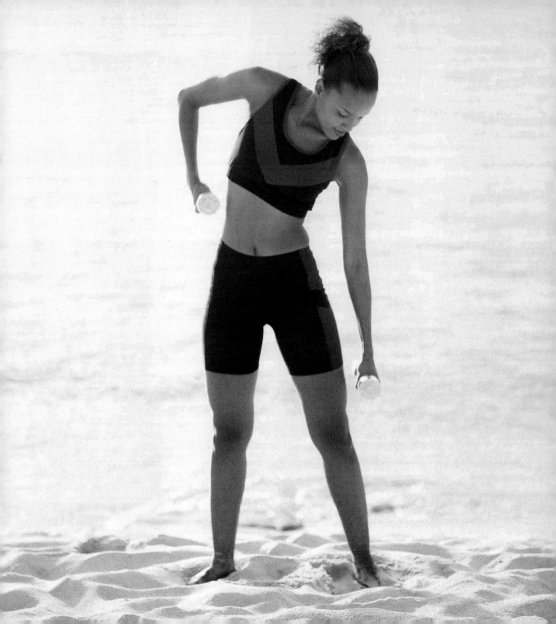

applying Zen

Although everything I have written so far on the subject of strength training has been negative, I am in fact an ardent supporter. Weight-training is one of the most powerful techniques I know to achieve measurable results. Although it is practiced mainly by men, it can be used to great effect by women. In order to build mass, the basic means is to train heavy/slow/few (heavy weights, slow reps), while to tone and develop endurance, train light/fast/many.

What I object to is how weight training is misused through ignorance and poor teaching. At present, anyone going to a gym thinks that weight-training is straightforward, and that they do not need any special instruction. No one would dream of picking up techniques such as swimming, karate, or aerobics without consulting a qualified instructor.

One possible solution to the misuses and abuses of strength training that I have described, would be the application of the principles of Zen, just as they were applied to archery and fencing in Medieval Japan, giving us the arts of kyudo and kendo. This is not as absurd as it sounds. The ritualization of the exercises would ensure their correct performance, while the spiritual discipline would ensure that the worst excesses of the sport would be avoided.

Conversely, I have always been intrigued by the thought that the strength trainer has already acquired many of the skills needed to progress in the study of Zen—the discipline and concentration necessary to study Zen techniques and to perform them correctly.

Conventional recommendations

for strength training with weights are to train the major muscle groups (legs, back, chest, shoulders, arms, and abdominal muscles) two to three times a week, with three sets of ten repetitions per exercise.

Recent research into weight-training, however, has shown that for beginners there is an advantage in performing just one set of each exercise rather than the conventionally prescribed two or three. It has been shown that beginners following light training schedules make faster gains that a more hard-working control group.

Strength training is particularly recommended for people in their fifties and beyond to make up for muscle wastage (the loss of muscle fibers that occurs with age), and to ameliorate several degenerative conditions, such osteoporosis and certain forms of arthritis.

strength-training

Lifting a weight from the floor

One of the most common causes of traumatic injury is improper lifting technique. The object does not even need to be particularly heavy, as the strain it causes to the musculature is increased by its position at the end of the arm.

When picking up a load from floor level, such as a box:

- Bend the knees to lower your entire body to be level with the object to be lifted.
- With your elbows bent, and the object securely held as close to your body as is practical, push up using the strength in your thighs.

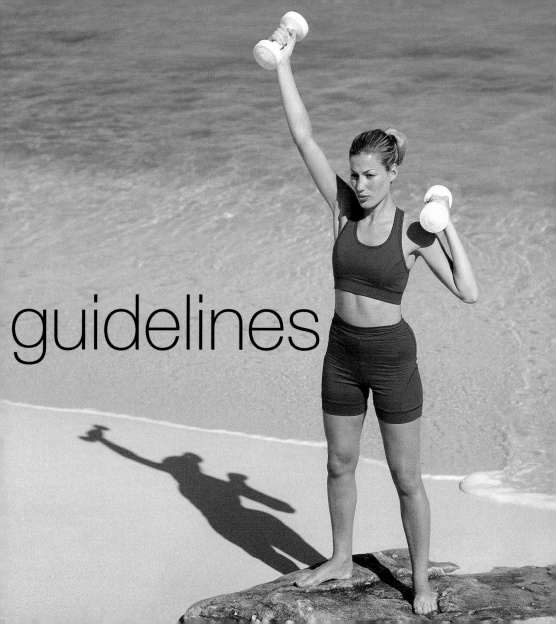

guidelines

working out your 1RM
(One Repetition Maximum)

Your 1RM represents the maximum amount of weight you can lift in one repetition on a given exercise. As this is potentially a dangerous procedure, it is recommended that you perform this test with a qualified instructor or an experienced weight-trainer. If you are attempting this on your own, only use weight-training machines.

Follow the instructions for the weight exercises given below, setting the load on a machine to a weight you can only lift once. If you have never weight trained before, it may take several attempts before you reach the desired weight. The following table gives suggested beginners' starting weights to test for 1RM for the main weight-training exercises.

	Men	Women
Bench press	110lb	65lb
Leg press	110lb	65lb
Lat pulldown	65lb	45lb
Biceps curl	20lb	10lb
Triceps press	20lb	10lb
Shoulder press	20lb	10lb

Once you have determined your 1RM for the major weight-training exercises, you will be able to decide the level of your training in terms of the percentage of your 1RM. In general, training close to your 1RM (70–99 percent) will build muscle mass, while training at the lower range of your 1RM (1–50 percent) will develop tone and endurance. Training in the midzone, will develop a combination of the two. A word of caution: If you have never weight trained before, consult a physician before beginning your training program.

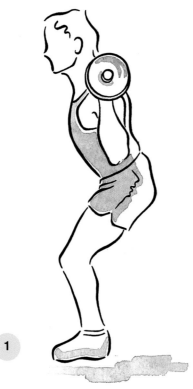

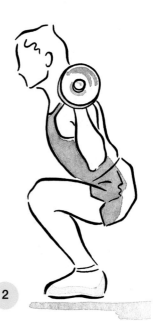

weight-assisted workout
(free weights)

squat (thighs and hips)

1 With a weighted barbell resting on your shoulders, stand with your feet slightly wider than shoulder-width apart, and parallel or slightly turned out, as is most comfortable.

2 Breathe out, and without leaning forward or raising your feet off the ground (rest your heels on a plank or weight plate if you have a tendency to raise your feet), bend your knees and lower your body until your thighs are parallel with the ground. Hold momentarily and breathe in as you return to the starting position.

Beginner:
1 set, 10 repetitions, 20–30% 1RM
Intermediate:
2 sets, 8–12 repetitions, 40–60% 1RM

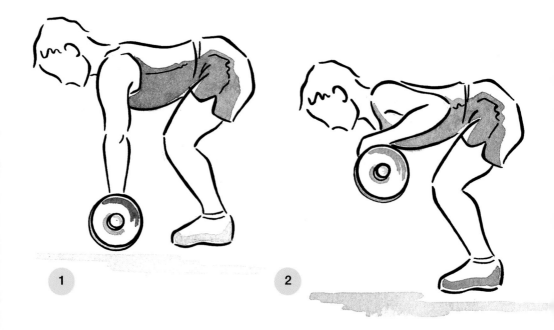

bent-over row (back and biceps)

1 Stand with your legs slightly more than shoulder-width apart. Keeping your knees bent, and your back flat, hold a weighted barbell at arms' length with your hands in a shoulder-width overhand grip.

2 Breathe in as you raise the barbell smoothly until it touches your ribcage. Hold momentarily, and breathe out as you lower the weight smoothly without letting it drop.

Beginner:
   1 set, 10 repetitions, 20–30% 1RM
Intermediate:
   2 sets, 8–12 repetitions, 40–60% 1RM

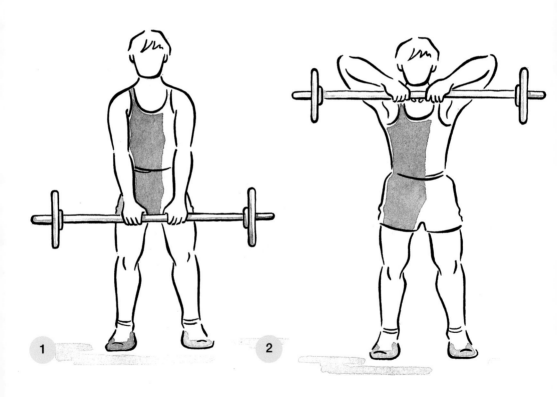

upright row
(upper back and shoulders)

1 Stand with your feet shoulder-width apart. Hold a weighted barbell with a narrow
   overhand grip (hands together or no more than four inches apart).

2 Breathe in and raise the bar to your chin by following the line of your body
   (i.e., do not swing out the bar). Keep your elbows as high as possible.
   Hold momentarily before you lower the bar.

Beginner:
   1 set, 10 repetitions, 20–30% 1RM
Intermediate:
   2 sets, 8–12 repetitions, 40–60% 1RM

bench press (chest and triceps)

1 Lying on a bench press, with your head and back flat on the bench and your feet flat on the ground, hold the bar with a wider than shoulder-width grip.

2 Lift the barbell off the rack, breathe out as you lower the bar to your chest, touching your chest lightly at the level of your nipples. Pause momentarily, and breathe in as you raise the barbell to arms' length.

Beginner:
   1 set, 10 repetitions, 20–30% 1RM
Intermediate:
   2 sets, 8–12 repetitions, 40–60% 1RM

shoulder press (shoulders)

1 Stand with your feet shoulder-width apart with a weighted barbell on your shoulders as in the squat. Do not lean back during this exercise (correct any tendency to do so by performing the press seated with your back supported).

2 Breathe in and press the bar up to arms' length. Hold for a moment, and breathe out and lower slowly to your shoulders.

Beginner:

   1 set, 10 repetitions, 20–30% 1RM

Intermediate:

   2 sets, 8–12 repetitions, 40–60% 1RM

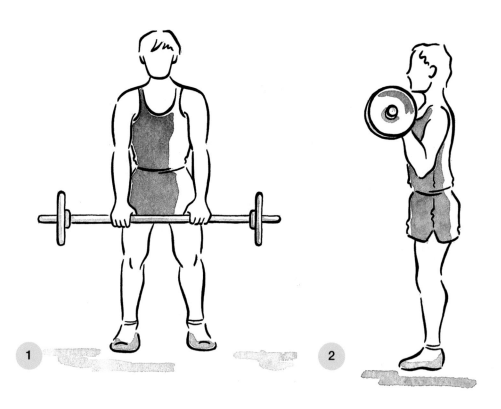

arm curl (biceps)

1 Stand with your feet shoulder-width apart. Hold a weighted barbell at arms'
   length with an underhand grip, so that your arms are in contact with your sides.
2 Breathe in and raise the bar, hinging from the elbow and trying not to move
   the upper arms, until the bar reaches the chest. Hold for a moment,
   then breathe out as you lower the bar.

Beginner:
   1 set, 12 repetitions 20–30% 1RM
Intermediate:
   2 sets, 12–15 repetitions, 40–60% 1RM

triceps press (triceps)

1   Stand with your feet shoulder-width apart holding a light barbell at
    arms' length with a shoulder-width overhand grip.
2   Breathe out as you bend your elbows, lowering the weight behind
    your head. Try to keep the upper arms still, breathe in, and raise the barbell.

Beginner:
   1 set, 12 repetitions, 20–30% 1RM
Intermediate:
   2 set, 12–15 repetitions, 40–60% 1RM

calf raise (calf)

1 Stand with your feet shoulder-width apart with a weighted barbell on your shoulders.

2 Raise yourself onto tiptoe and then lower yourself. Move slowly and smoothly.

Beginner:

1 set, 20 repetitions, 20–30% 1RM

Intermediate:

2 sets, 20–25 repetitions, 40–60% 1RM

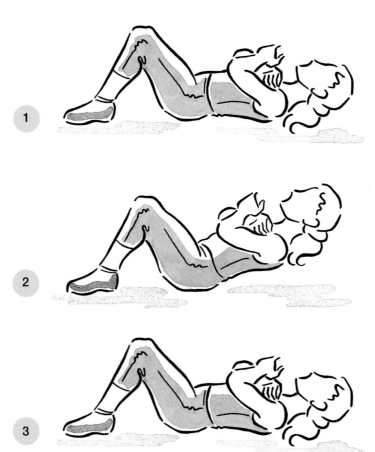

crunch (upper abdominals)

1 Lie on the floor, with your knees bent and your arms crossed on your chest.

2 Contract your stomach muscles, imagining that you are pulling up from them to lift your upper back and head from the mat. Do not lead with your head or shoulders. Move slowly and smoothly without jerking.

3 Hold momentarily, and then lower your body.

Beginner:

2 sets, 20 repetitions

Intermediate:

3–5 sets, 20–25 repetitions

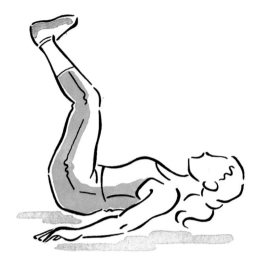

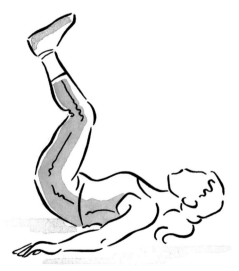

reverse crunch (lower abdominals)

1 Lie on your back. Raise your legs, keeping them bent at the knees or holding them straight up.

2 Contract your abdominal muscles and raise your buttocks off the floor. Do not exaggerate the movements or hurl yourself in the air. Keep the movement slow and smooth.

Beginner:
   2 sets, 20 repetitions
Intermediate:
   3–5 sets, 20–25 repetitions

oblique
crunch (sides)

1 Lie on the floor as in the crunch.

2 Instead of raising your body forward, raise alternately to the right and left.

Beginner:

2 sets, 20 repetitions (each side)

Intermediate:

3-5 sets, 20–25 repetitions (each side)

back raise
(lower back)

1 Lie on your stomach with your arms linked behind your back.
2 Contract the muscles in your lower back, and pull your chest and head off the mat. Do not lead with your head or jerk your head back.

Beginner:
  2 sets, 20 repetitions
Intermediate:
  3–5 sets, 20–25 repetitions

chapter 7

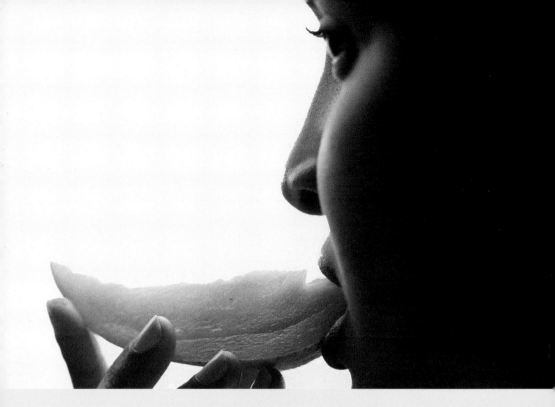

right livelihood: diet and self-image

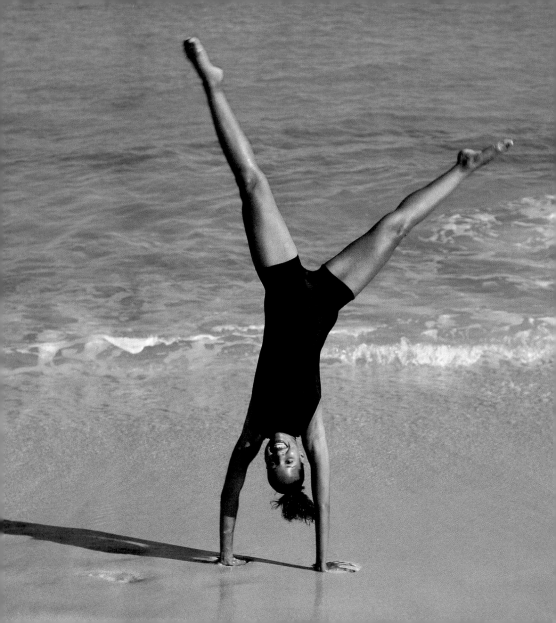

Meditation: "Get rid of the self, and act from the Self!"—Zen saying

In the Buddhist view of human nature, until we enter the path of liberation, we are all addicts hooked on the pleasures that the world has to offer: food, sex, wealth, power, and fame. Although our dependence may not be as severe and self-destructive as, say, the alcoholic's or the drug addict's, the difference is only one of degree. The more single-mindedly we pursue material and sensual satisfaction, the more it seems to elude us, until our failure plunges us into a melancholia of despair.

just desserts

My family and some of our friends
were sitting down to a birthday meal at an
expensive restaurant. It was a scene that could take place
anywhere in the developed world. My brother and I, aged ten and
twelve, were excited by our first grown-up meal out but visibly
uncomfortable in the formal clothes we rarely wore. But this was the kind of
establishment that insists that all "gentlemen" wear a shirt, necktie, and jacket. We
had eaten our starters and main courses, and were waiting for our desserts.
"And what would you like for dessert?" my mother asked. I looked greedily down the
menu. "A banana-split," I reply after ruling out the less tempting offerings and imagining the
gooey concoction of ice cream, fruit, and sauce, topped with whipped cream.
My mother frowned. "Wouldn't you prefer some fruit salad like your brother?" she asked. She is
worried because I had been putting on weight since she divorced my father a year earlier. There
are two distinct physical types in my family. My father's side has the dark hair and skin, short to
medium stature, and wiry frames that are associated with Latin ancestry; while my mother's side
has northern European characteristics: they are taller, stockier, blondes and redheads. Their
attitude about food (and life generally) mirrors their physiques, though in a classic chicken-
and-egg scenario, it is difficult to say which is the cause and which the result.
Although both sides produce slim children and adolescents, the dark side are more
puritanical in their habits. They eat plain food and drink only
on special occasions (or not at all in my father's case). The
fair side, who could be described as bon vivants,
uncork a bottle and bake muffins and cookies
at the slightest excuse.

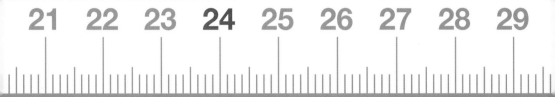

The results are plain to see: by the time they reach middle age, my paternal kin are physically unchanged, while the maternal kin has let out its communal belt by several notches. The latter have reduced their life expectancy by a few years, but there is nothing more sinister in the family's attitude to food than overindulgence. They are typical of the majority of the 50 percent of British and Americans who are now considered overweight. They are guilty of the three deadly sins against current thinking on health and fitness. They do not know what constitutes a balanced diet (IGNORANCE), do not do enough physical exercise (SLOTH), and they let themselves be tempted by the high-fat, high-sugar foods that are all around us (GREED). In my case, however, greed, sloth, and ignorance were not the causes of my incipient weight

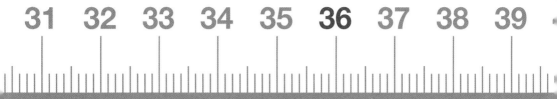

problem. When I was nine, my parents' marriage broke down, and the fallout at home was pretty distressing. I can only imagine that I tried to escape the stress of the situation through one of the few pleasures open to children: food. Over a period of years I was eating more calories than I was using up, and ironically, it was only by the time my parents had divorced, that it began to be noticeable. It is unfortunate that the time lag built into the process meant that I was going to experience the physical (and social) consequences of my parents' breakup well after the event had taken place.

My stepfather, who, I must stress, is a very kind and loving man, has been good-naturedly ignoring us children for most of the meal, and talking to his adult guests, intervened. "Let him have what he wants."

I get my banana split, and it is stickier and sweeter than I had imagined. I dispatch it so quickly that my dish is empty before everyone at the table has been served their own desserts. I do not so much enjoy my food as inhale it. I have not savored the different elements of the banana split, merely given my taste buds a short-lived taste rush, which does not give them a chance to be sated, I have given my bloodstream an equally short-lived sugar high.

Although my stepfather has a grown-up son of his own, he has not been in close contact with children for more than twenty years. He studies me as if I was the representative of an interesting, yet totally alien, species.

"Would you like another one?" he asks.

"Oh, yes please," I reply, agog that an adult is offering more of what I crave. My horrified mother looks imploringly at us. But her son is determined to have his second dessert, and her husband is determined to carry out his psychological experiment: How many banana splits can a boy of ten eat before he is sick?

The second dessert is ordered. By this time everyone at the table has finished their own desserts. My older brother has decided that I do not exist and is pointedly looking away to the side, and the adults are having coffee; their attentions, however, are riveted by the second banana split that is brought in on a silver platter and placed in front of me.

dieting

Looking back on this period with the hindsight of thirty years' experience, it is obvious to me that I was "comfort eating," but at the time, I was not aware that anything out of the ordinary was going on. The process was so gradual, and its consequences did not become fully apparent until after the divorce had long been settled.

When the summer holidays came around the year of my thirteenth birthday, I decided to lose the excess weight. I was never bullied at school for being fat, but there are many more subtle ways that children make each other feel different and ill at ease. With my mother's help, I opted for a sensible calorie-controlled diet.

The one-thousand-calorie-a-day diet was then in vogue. Although one thousand calories is much too low for a growing child, one of the diet's strong points is that it does not limit you in your choice of foods, but discourages you from "blowing" your daily allowance on calorie-rich, high-fat and high-sugar foods. I doubt if I ever stuck to the limit of one thousand calories.

I lived on a diet of seafood, fish, fresh fruit and vegetables, and French bread, thus significantly reducing the excess fats and sugars in my diet, but without reducing the proteins, complex carbohydrates, and essential nutrients—vitamins and minerals—that I needed as a growing adolescent.

I dieted and lost weight, but I did so safely. At the same time, I increased the amount of exercise I did by swimming out to a line of buoys about three hundred yards out to sea several times a day. After two months of this regime, I had lost the excess twenty pounds I was carrying.

I arrived back at school in the fall of that year, with a much trimmer and more fashionable figure. My mother, to congratulate me on my success, bought me a particularly trendy shirt, which I proudly wore on my first day of classes. I bumped into friends, enjoying their yelps of surprise and wallowing in their praise. Later that afternoon came the ultimate high school accolade: I was invited to my first teen party by one of the popular girls.

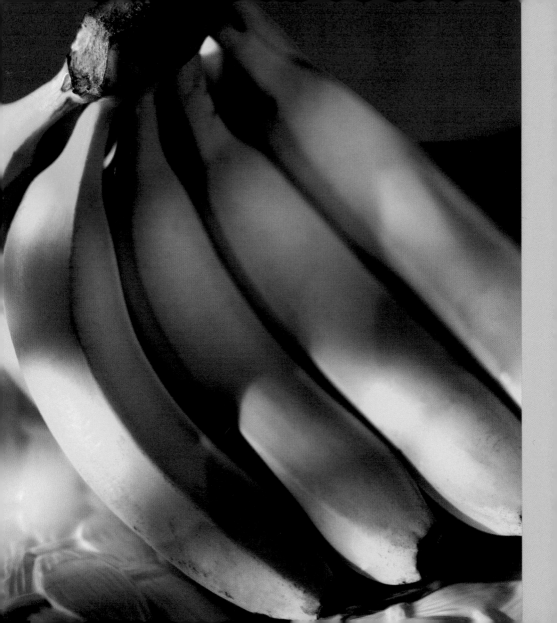

As for my stepfather's banana split experiment, you can no doubt imagine the result. The third dessert arrived. It went, not surprisingly, the same way as the first two, and almost as fast. What he had failed to take into account in his equation was the greed and eating capacity of a ten-year-old boy. I finished the third banana split, and looked up at him to see if any more were forthcoming. He looked away and called for the check. I think it was the first time he had had to admit defeat in a very long time.

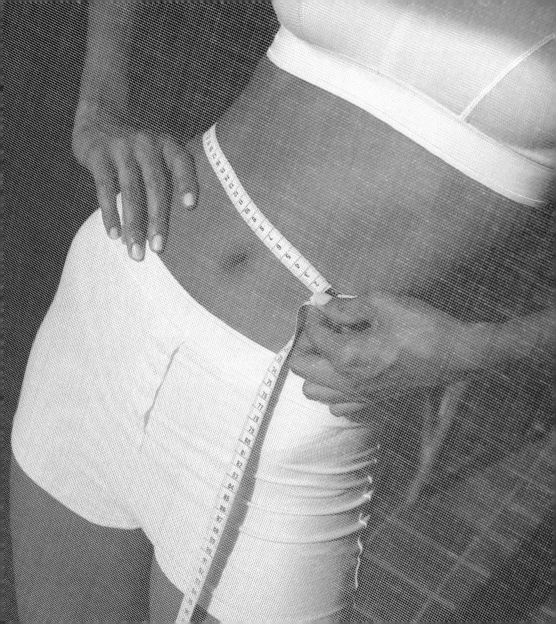

Starvation dieting, as we all now know, is counterproductive, as it slows the metabolism down, and leads to weight gain in the long run. There is only one way to reduce excess body fat safely and permanently (see pages 268–276). The novelty diets that appear in books or magazines are at best only temporarily effective because they alter, but do not change, your eating habits, and at worst are dangerous because they make you lose weight in a way that damages your body by depriving it of essential nutrients. One such diet is the recent zero-carbohydrate weight-loss program, which deprives your body of its natural fuel, and encourages you to eat high-fat foods that damage your cardiovascular health.

Following a sensible eating plan to reduce weight may not reap instant results, but the controlled, healthy approach will reap greater long-term benefits and will enable you to maintain your ideal weight. Make yourself aware of the nutritional value of foods— which food products provide you with the

A sensible diet

most protein, iron, and fiber—and adapt these according to where you are in your life cycle. For instance a woman in her twenties and thirties is still building bones and needs to make sure she has plenty of calcium in her diet to prevent the onset of osteoporosis in later life.

Although I suffered from an "eating disorder" as a child, its long-term effects have been surprisingly benign for my general health. I resolved the issue in time, before being fat could itself become a health problem or a social issue. As I grew older, I retained a much higher awareness of health and fitness issues concerning nutrition than my peers and, though my exercise habits have sometimes verged on the obsessive, as a whole, I can say that my sense of well-being has definitely benefited. Without a doubt the most valuable insight I got from the experience, however, was the understanding that with the correct motivation and knowledge, we all have the ability to effect real change in ourselves.

Chinese water torture

I also count myself very fortunate that food was my most dangerous addiction. Had I been a little older at the time of my parents' divorce, I might have been tempted to resort to more dangerous substances, such as alcohol or drugs. As it was, when the moment came, several years later, when I was exposed to alcohol, my "addictive moment" had passed. I sampled what was offered, found that alcohol provided a transient form of pleasure, but decided that the cost that was rarely, if ever, worth paying.

One of the most common, yet, even now, the least recognized form of substance abuse is alcohol dependency. Masked by social acceptance of alcohol, alcoholism can remain hidden for decades—even from the drinker himself. I have lost two close friends to alcohol—not because they died from one of the many alcohol-related illnesses, but because of the slow and seemingly inexorable change in their personalities. The first was the "life and soul of the party"—a bubbling extrovert who began as a social drinker. But the alcohol that she increasingly counted on to allow her to sparkle at social gatherings finally plunged her into suicidal depression, because the prolonged use of large doses of alcohol is a strong depressant. The second was a shy and introverted young man. He, too, drank to overcome low self-esteem, but soon he became trapped in a vicious circle in which his failure to stop drinking was seen as further confirmation of his worthlessness.

To my knowledge both are still alive and still drinkers, because alcohol is a slow and insidious killer that works one drop at a time like Chinese water torture. So were they "addictive personalities" who could not help themselves? They would like to believe so, and thus deny their own responsibility for their actions.

Buddhism, however, teaches us that we are the complete masters of our fate. There is no permanent personality, so there can be no "addictive" or "non-addictive" personalities. I believe that we all have our "addictive moments," as I did when I was an unhappy child. But the unhappy child grows up, so why continue to be the child when you are now the adult?

smoking gun

I realized how powerful a chemical dependence could be when I wanted to give up smoking. I had started the habit as a teenager for the all the wrong social reasons. Nicotine is one of the most addictive substances known to man; it is said to be more addictive than heroin in that it takes only one cigarette to turn a nonsmoker into an addicted smoker. Fortunately, the addiction is also extremely short-lived.

When I confided in my first *t'ai chi* teacher that I wanted to stop smoking he asked me if I was really serious about stopping. I answered that I was.

Satisfied, he said, "If you follow my advice to the letter, you will be free of your addiction to cigarettes in three days." Three days, I thought to myself. The limitation on the period was reassuring. Smokers often put off quitting because they think that their craving for cigarettes will never leave them. In reality, the physical craving fades very quickly, leaving only the psychological addiction.

For the next three days I was to eat only apples and drink only apple juice and water. I asked him why apples. The pectin, which is a chemical in apples that helps jam set, he replied, would detoxify my system, and eliminate the craving for nicotine.

I do not know whether there is a scientific basis for this, but I can confirm that his advice worked. By day two, I was so hungry and obsessing so much about the food I was not eating, that my craving for nicotine went unnoticed. By day three, cleansed of my physical dependence on cigarettes, I had to deal with my psychological dependence, which was far more insidious. I found myself thinking that since I had given up smoking so easily, I could stop whenever I wanted, so one cigarette from time to time would not hurt. This was a lot harder to deal with than the hysterical, "If I don't have another cigarette I'll die!" which is triggered by the physical withdrawal from a powerfully addictive drug.

inner strength

Unfortunately, this was not quite the end of the story. Several years later, in a moment of crisis, I lapsed and started smoking again. I knew that I had stopped once before, and this knowledge somehow lulled me into a false sense of security. I could stop whenever I wanted, I reasoned. After one year had gone by and I was still smoking, I decided I must stop—this time, for good. In terms of health, there can be no greater threat than the diseases that are caused by cigarettes, from cancers of the lungs and throat, to emphysema, bronchitis, and heart disease.

In a sense, the first time I had tricked myself into stopping. I had borrowed another person's strength—in this case, my *t'ai chi* teacher's—and used my belief and trust in him and his miracle apple cure to quit instead of counting on my own strength. I knew that after three days, I would no longer be a smoker. In that period I would have quit nicotine "cold turkey," and there would be none of the drug left in my system. In a matter of weeks, in fact, I would no more be a smoker than people who had never smoked in their lives.

As for the psychological addiction, it was not a WWF match between "in the red corner, Eric, and in the blue corner, the reigning champion of the word, Mr Cigarette!" As soon as the addiction was no longer able to call upon external support (nicotine dependence), I was the only person giving it strength—it was only as strong as I cared to make it.

the Zen
eating plan?

The precepts of Zen Buddhism concerning diet and stimulants are brief. The domination of the body's cravings is taken for granted for the student entering the path of study, for the student will have to overcome far more difficult temptations as he advances. The rule that most Zen establishments follow is not unlike that of Western monasteries: food sustains the body of the student in training, and it should not be enjoyed in its own right. The diet is vegetarian, in accord with the ethical teachings of the Buddha concerning the sacredness of all life. The only stimulant allowed to students is strong green tea, to help them stay awake during long periods of meditation.

Zen does not discriminate on the grounds of appearance or body size. On the contrary, personal vanity belongs to that class of illusions about the self that ensnares humans and makes them unhappy. But a dependence on food, like an addiction to any kind of drug—legal or illegal—will present a very real obstacle to study and must be dealt with first. Zen , however, is not a health cure or a diet aid. It will teach that dependence on external stimuli impedes your progress, but it has no tricks or techniques that will help you control your weight. It is not to be co-opted like many other spiritual teachings to the whims of the diet industry to provide another hard-sell slogan "I shed the pounds with the Zen Eating Plan! Yours to own for just $9.99."

In the fight against addiction, Zen offers two very powerful weapons: zazen meditation, which pacifies the troubled mind and gradually cuts the links that bind you to the external world (see Chapter 8), and the certainty that, no matter who we are, we are capable of change.

nutrition
guidelines

On the physical level, weight control is simply a question of supply and demand. Eat too much (oversupply) and you gain weight, eat too little (under-supply) and you lose weight. Most people, however, are ignorant of how much food (usually expressed in calories) they need to eat per day. The tables and equations given on the following pages will allow you to work out your daily calorie expenditure, and with the help of a calorie guide you can calculate how close you are to your optimum intake at present.

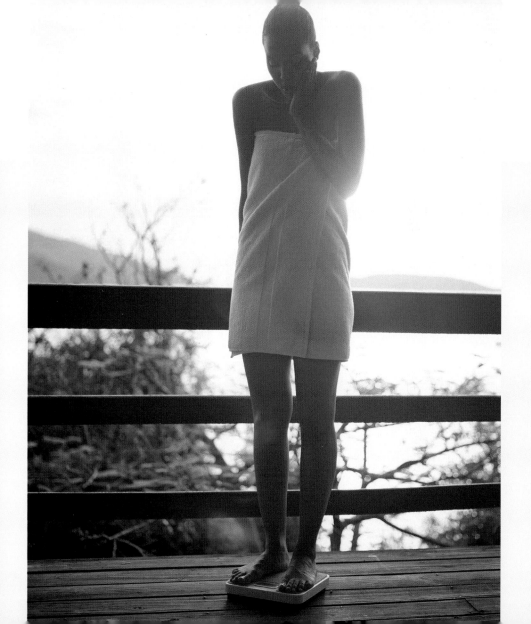

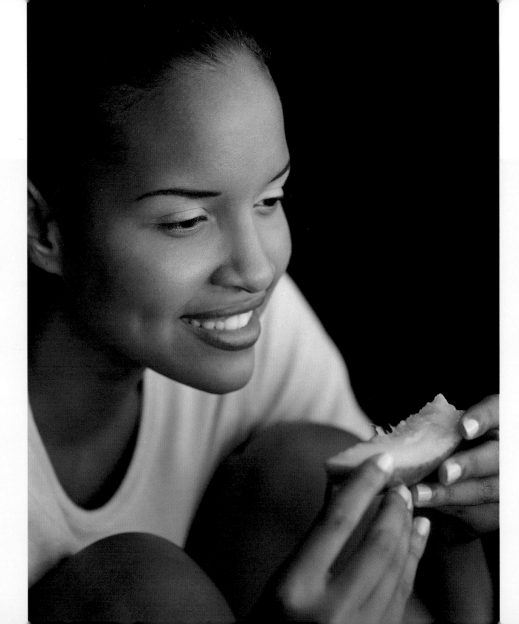

Working out your
Base Metabolic Rate (BMR)

Your BMR is the amount of energy, expressed in terms of calories, your body uses up in twenty-four hours for essential activities such as breathing, digesting food, etc., but excluding any physical activity.

Women

665 + (9.56 x weight in kg) + (1.85 x height in cm) - (4.68 x age)*

Example: A 20-year-old woman, 160 cm (5 ft 2 in) tall, weighing 60 kg (132 lb)

665 + (9.56 x 60) + (1.85 x 160) - (4.68 x 20) = 1441 calories

Men

66.5 + (13.8 x weight in kg) + (5 x height in cm) - (6.76 x age)*

Example: A 40-year-old man, 180 cm (5 ft 9 in) tall, weighing 80 kg (176 lb)

66.5 + (13.8 x 80) + (5 x 180) - (6.76 x 44) = 2069 calories

* Complete the calculations in the parentheses then add and subtract as required.

calorie audit

1 To work out how many calories you use in one twenty-four-hour period, follow these steps. First break down your day in terms of activities and grade them according to the following table:

Activity as multiple of BMR

Activity	BMR x
Sleeping, lying down	1.0
Very light (seated and standing activities, such as driving, working at a desk, typing)	1.5
Light (Walking slowly on a level surface, housework, sports such as golf and bowling)	2.5
Moderate (Walking briskly, gardening, medium intensity sports such as tennis)	5.0
Heavy (Walking uphill with a load, manual labor, high-intensity sports such as triathlon)	7.0

2 This will give you this kind of breakdown for your daily activities. Example:

Activity	duration	rating
Sleeping	8 hours	x 1.0
Commuting	1 hour	x 1.5
Working	8 hours	x 1.5
Gym session	1 hour	x 5.0
Commuting	1 hour	x 1.5
Evening activities	5 hours	x 1.5

3 Multiply the hours you spend doing each activity by the rating, add them up, and then divide by twenty-four to derive your average daily energy expenditure rate.

8 x 1.0 = 8

1 x 1.5 = 1.5

8 x 1.5 = 12

1 x 5   = 5

1 x 1.5 = 1.5

5 x 1.5 = 7.5

Total: 35.5 ÷ 24 = 1.47

4 Finally, multiply your average daily expenditure rate by your BMR to give you your total calorie expenditure. For example, for someone with a BMR of 1441:

1441 x 1.47 = 2118 calories/day

weight-loss target

A pound of body fat is 3,500 calories. Multiply the number of pounds you wish to lose by this figure. For example, a 185-pound man wishing to lose 20 pounds will have to lose 70,000 calories. A realistic target for weight loss is one pound of fat per week, so the daily target in calorie reduction is 3500 ÷ 7 = 500 calories per day.

Remember, if you are trying to lose weight, set yourself realistic targets and follow these guidelines.

- Lose no more than one pound per week.
- Do not reduce your daily calorie intake by more than 500 calories and never drop below 1,500 cals/day.
- Maintain balanced diet: 60 percent carbohydrates, 10–20 percent proteins, and 10–20 percent fats (i.e., do not cut out one food group, such as carbohydrates, fats, or proteins).
- If possible, increase the amount of physical activity in your daily routine.

the
Mediterranean diet

Eating the right number of calories will help you control your weight, but it does not mean that you will be eating healthily. In recent years, doctors have come to recognize that there is one diet that meets practically all the guidelines for healthy eating—that of the countries of the Mediterranean, particularly Italy and Spain. Here are the basic elements of the diet:

- Ideal balance of food groups (carbohydrates: 60 percent, proteins: 10 percent, fats: 30 percent)
- High in complex carbohydrates (pasta, rice, bread, etc.) for energy
- Low in saturated fats
- Low in dairy products
- Low in refined sugars
- Use of monounsaturated olive oil (olic acid reduces total and bad cholesterol and increases good cholesterol)
- High in fresh fruits and vegetables, which provide antioxidants to eliminate free radicals
- Inclusion of red wine which contains antioxidant compounds (restrict to a maximum of two small glasses a day, as alcohol is high in empty calories)

If you're a smoker and have decided to quit, set the date that you are going to stop.

1 Remove all smoking materials and reminders of smoking the night before you go to bed.

2 Purchase a sufficient supply of apples, apple juice, and water to last you a three-day period.

3 You may wish to prepare the apple in a variety of ways to alleviate the monotony of the diet. Preparation methods include sliced apple salads, baked apples, stewed and puréed apples, etc. In all cases leave the skin on the fruit.

4 As you will not be eating your usual diet, and one which is deficient in carbohydrates, fats, and proteins, do not plan to do any exercise or hard manual labor during the three-day period. Use it to catch up on reading, writing, or merely rest and relaxation.

stop smoking apple detox

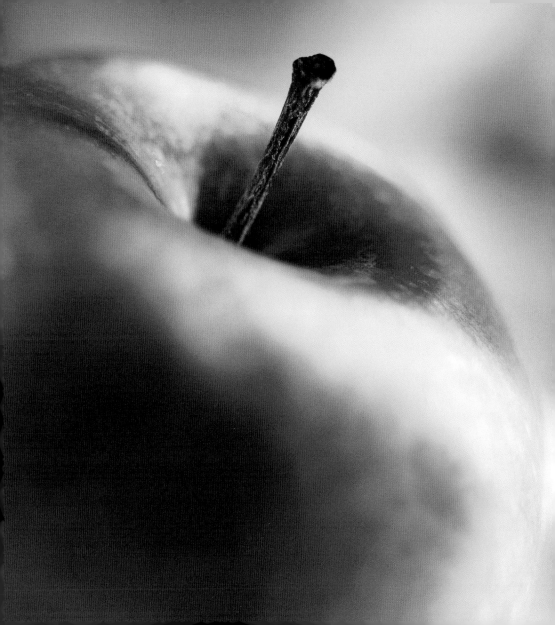

chapter 8

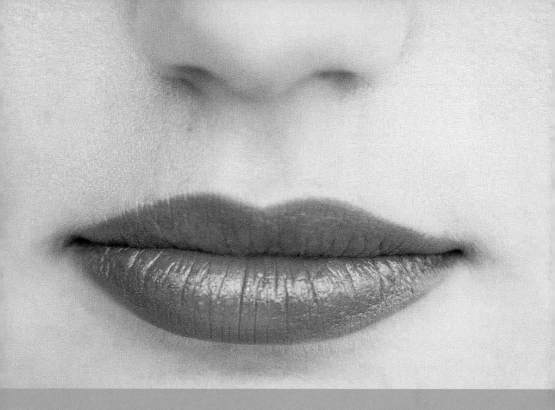

right concentration: stress

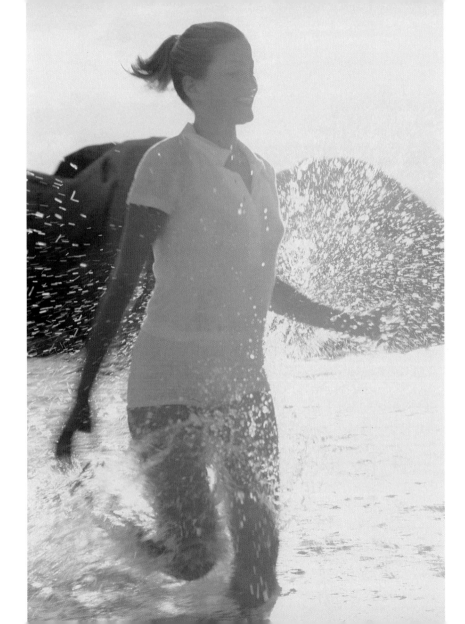

Meditation: "I'm the greatest." —Mohammad Ali (Cassius Clay)

Stress is fast becoming the number one health problem in the developed world, and the major obstacle to maintaining our sense of well-being. Although present day stress has mental not physical causes, it is known to trigger a set of responses in the body that contribute to a wide range of physical ailments. Unfortunately, the conventional Western dualistic view that separates the mind from the body leaves us poorly prepared to deal with stress-related symptoms. And although there is a growing awareness of the need to be physically fit, there is too little recognition of the mental preparations we need to make in order to deal with stress and maintain a positive outlook on life.

depression
depression
depression
depression
depression
depression

Bastille Day 1992 was not a good day for me. Two weeks after I had seen my mother die of cancer at the Houston Medical Center, my partner of six years' standing announced the end of our relationship. At work, I had just completed a major, two-year project, the translation and editing of a major work of Japanese literature, which put a large question mark over my future career. At that moment, it seemed that everything that could go wrong with my life had gone wrong.

Although I had hitherto always been able to control stress with regular exercise and occasional meditation, the strain of my mother's final illness and the recent pressure of work had left me suffering the classic symptoms of stress: depression, moodiness, insomnia, headaches, lack of appetite, and low energy levels. I was in no doubt about the nature of my condition, but I was already losing the battle. It was at that moment that my partner decided to deliver the coup de grâce. The closest I can come to a description of what I felt at that moment was that I no longer wanted to exist. There was no place I wanted to be, no person I wanted to be with, and nothing that I wanted to do.

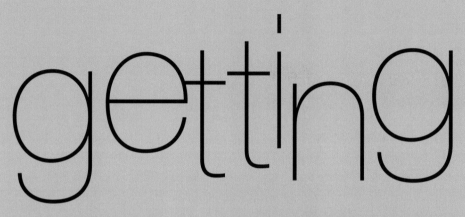

getting

I decided without the slightest qualm or hesitation that what I needed to do was to get so drunk that I would no longer be conscious of the pain and disappointment. It was a crude attempt at sedation, but after a slightly false start, it did work.

I went to a bar I sometimes frequented after work with colleagues and ordered a double vodka, much to the surprise of the bartender who was more accustomed to serving me diet cola or orange juice.

Soon I was on my third vodka. As expected, I had bypassed the sense of euphoria that can accompany early stages of drinking, but the pain was definitely dulling. It was at this particular moment, much to my later shame, that I got into a fight.

In every other respect a model establishment, this particular bar was frequented by a sad and absurd young man who, regardless of what you were doing at the time, would come up to you and attempt to begin a conversation. I have no doubt that he did it out of

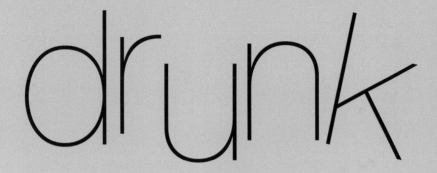

drunk

loneliness, and that he did not entirely deserve what was coming to him. The few patrons I knew in the bar could tell something was up and were leaving me alone, but the sad young man blithely came up to me and began his absurd chatter. However, instead of my usual amused response, what he got was a very curt and very clear instruction to get lost, couched in very unliterary language.

He stood with his mouth gaping for a moment. Confused and angry, he threw his drink at me—fortunately, it was only mineral water. I do not know if the bartender or the other customers ducked at this point in good Hollywood-movie style, but I would not have liked to see the look on my face. I did not shout or strike out at him. Unnaturally calm, I stood up and picked him up by his jacket collar and belt and, as if he weighed no more than a child. Oblivious to his blows and kicks, I carried him to the door, which I pushed open with my foot, and I threw him with some force out onto the sidewalk.

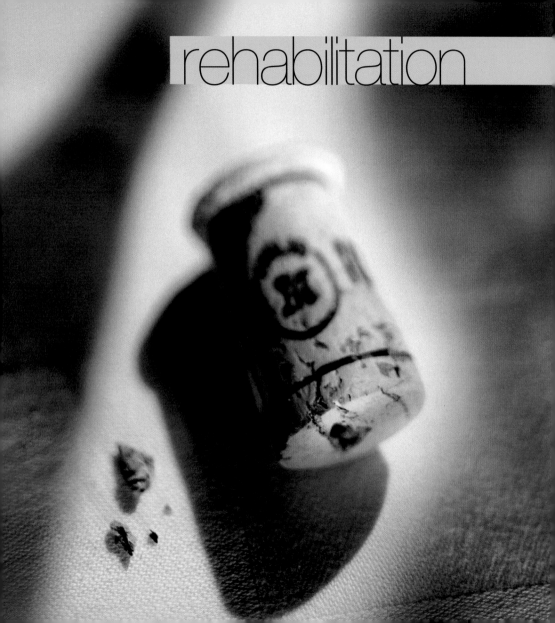

rehabilitation

I must repeat that I deplore what I did, but the sense of physical release was tremendous. I had not felt like exercising for over a week, having flown back from my mother's deathbed, and the physical tension had locked into my upper back, neck, shoulders, and chest. Physically liberated, but mentally unchanged, I went back to my seat at the bar and ordered another drink.

The bartender put another double in front of me. "On the house," he said when I tried to pay for it. "We've all been wanting to do that." Then he kept on serving me until I found the oblivion I was craving, which as a light drinker, came a few drinks later. I was put into a cab and sent home. I slept right through the next day, catching up on a lot of missed sleep. This continued the process of physical relaxation started by my impromptu exercise in the bar the night before. Fortunately, I also managed to sleep right through my hangover, and I awoke in the evening feeling disoriented but in a slightly improved state of mind.

I got on the phone to my closest friends, who were both then working on the other side of the world. It was good to hear the voices of people who really cared for me. They knew that I would never do anything "silly," and try to hurt myself (after I had told them what I had done in the bar, they were more concerned for any victims that might be strewn in my path!). The unquestioning emotional support, totally devoid of pity or panic, was the third phase in the process of my recovery.

A few days later, I got a call from one of my friends who had not heard of my recent troubles. He was the one looking for company and comfort, as he had just gone through a painful divorce. He was about to leave for a vacation in Australia, and, in one of those wonderful moments of marvelous coincidence, invited me to join him. I phoned the office, telling them I was taking a couple of weeks off and went to complete the process of my physical and mental recovery.

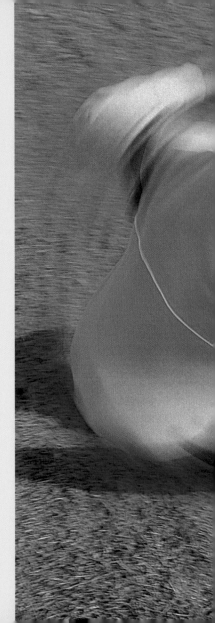

four-step plan

I was suffering from reactive depression, that is, one caused by events in the real world; in this case, the death of a parent and the end of a relationship. The steps I took, although unorthodox, were fortuitously exactly the ones I needed to initiate the lengthy process of recovery.

1 The alcohol provided a desensitizing sedative by shutting me down and allowing me to sleep. Had I gone to a doctor, he would have prescribed valium, or a similar tranquilizer, which would have had the same effect.

2 The fight provided a much needed physical release.

3 I obtained counseling and emotional support from friends.

4 The holiday temporarily removed me from the stresses of my work and home environment.

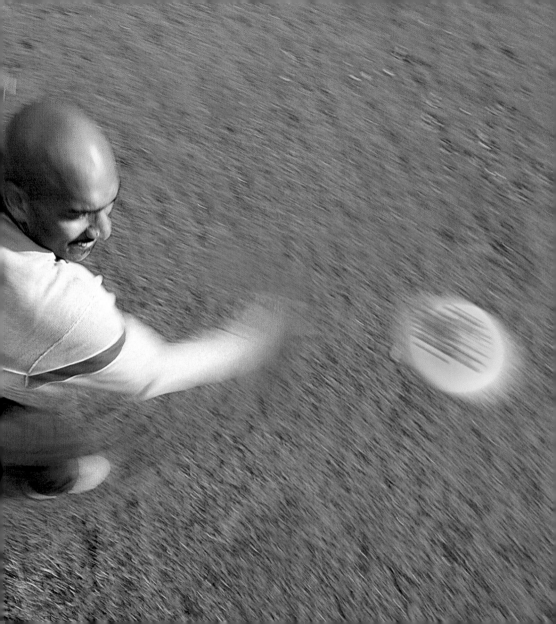

stress

The story above is an example of extreme stress, and no matter how well prepared I was, I do not think that I could have reacted any differently. Fortunately, although it may take years to deal fully with the grief of losing a parent or divorcing a spouse, the initial shock passes quickly. It is much more difficult and damaging to deal with the type of stress that does not have such immediately recognizable causes. Stress can manifest itself in a wide range of physical and mental symptoms (see the following pages), which are not always recognized for what they are.

In the opening meditation of this book we saw that our ancestors were exposed to high degrees of physical stress from the environment, but the stress we experience is completely different. The physical stress on our bodies comes from pollution and from excesses such as obesity and its related illnesses. Far more significant is the mental stress that begins for many of us in childhood, with the competition to pass exams to enter the best school, and continues into adulthood, as we are expected to succeed on our chosen career paths.

As a natural consequence of our failure to recognize stress-related symptoms, it comes as no surprise that we are not taught the techniques to overcome mental stress. Listed in the following table are some of the most common mental and physical responses to stress and their effects on the mind and body.

stress: responses and their effects

Physiological Responses

Epinephrin is released into bloodstream

Heart rate and blood preasure increase

Glycogen released by liver; blood sugar and cholesterol increases

Faster breathing and higher base metabolic rate

Muscular tension and increase of lactic acid

Gastric acid increases or decreases

Perspiration increases

Increased levels of cortisol; immune response suppressed

Emotional tension as mind is focused on crisis

Effects

High blood pressure, anxiety

Insomnia

High cholesterol

Hyperventilation, heart palpitations

Aches and pains

Indigestion, food intolerance, nausea

Skin rashes, eczema

Reduced immunity, minor ailments

Moodiness, depression

In moderation, stress is not only useful but necessary; it gives us the drive to improve our lives. It is only harmful when it is excessive, and there is no way to release it. Recognizing that we are suffering from stress is the first step, but dealing with it is not a simple matter. The most radical recommendation would be a complete change of lifestyle. Many men and women in the financial industry, one of the most stressful environments known to modern humans, can "burn out" in their thirties. If they are fortunate, they have earned enough money to be able to retire and change their lifestyles. They are the exception rather than the rule, because for many low-paid workers in stressful jobs, there is no such escape route.

assessing your lifestyle

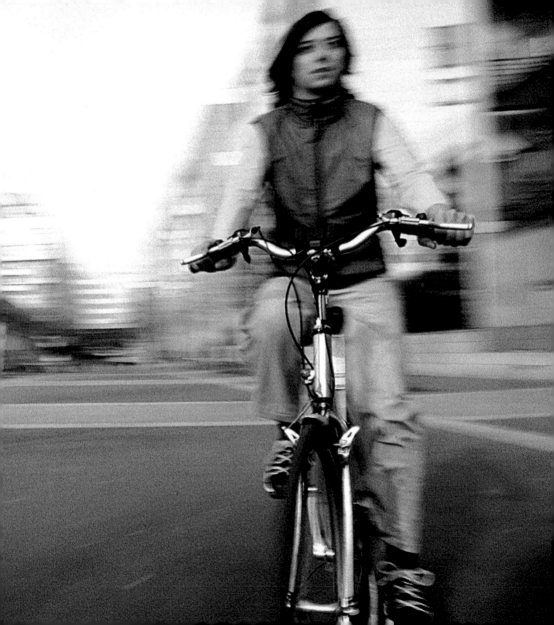

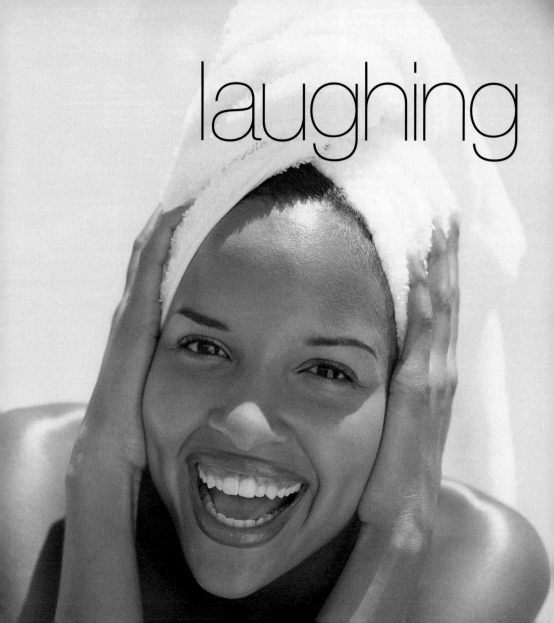

laughing

out loud

Another approach is to attack stress from the physical level. In addition to the techniques given in the practical section, there is something that is open to all of us that is a guaranteed cure for anxiety—laughter. While children laugh an average of three hundred times a day, in adulthood, this can be reduced to a mere fifty times a day. In *Laughter: The Best Medicine*, R. Holden describes the beneficial effects of laughter. The physical act of laughter makes you breathe more deeply, which not only relaxes the body, it also releases your body's own natural opiates, the endorphins, which naturally increase your sense of well-being. Finally, it raises the efficiency of the immune system, protecting you from disease.

However, laughter is of no avail when we have lost our sense of humor, as I did when I lost my will to live in 1992. I realized what a fragile thing the happiness that we make for ourselves in this life is, and how quickly it can be swept away by circumstances. Disappointment can easily turn us to bitterness and isolation, seeking solace in addiction to drink or drugs. Fortunately, I had already begun on the path, and Zen came to my rescue. Until then, I had merely used zazen (see pages 318–319) as a technique to control stress, creating pools of quietude in the torrent-like rush of life.

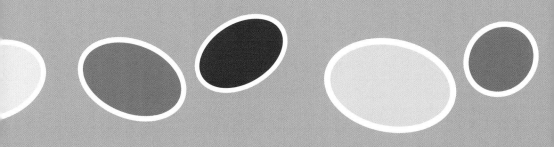

Zen and the art of well-being

I finally experienced firsthand the truth in the teachings of the Buddha. I had seen death at close hand and been given a direct intimation of my own passing. I come from the most successful material culture on earth, which can fulfill the hedonistic needs and sensual expectations of an unprecedented number of human beings, yet, in the end, I know that it will fail me. The first consolation of Zen has been the understanding of the human condition that it brings. But while it forces us to admit that we are not immortal, and that external reality can never satisfy us, Zen is not a negative, nihilistic philosophy. Liberated from our illusions, we are free to go forward to discover the true nature of well-being. But,

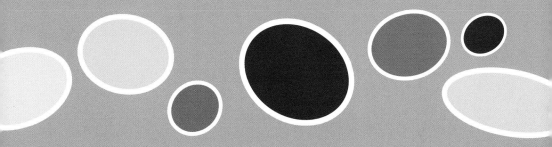

unlike our forebears, who had to cram everything into lives of forty years, we do not need to rush.

I am the first to admit that I have lived my life experiencing my senses to the fullest. I am not like that old hypocrite, Saint Augustine of Hippo, who lived the life of a sinner in his youth, repented and reformed when he became an old man, and preached restraint to the young. Zen does not deny the power of physical pleasure. Instead it recognizes it attractions, and advises its devotees to come to terms with sex—the red thread of passion—which will otherwise become an insurmountable obstacle in their path.

I may see the world exactly for what it is, without illusions or blinkers. I know that I will age, sicken, and die, as surely as I saw my mother die, but I am not morose or depressed. Nor am I content with throwing myself into a round of pleasures. In the practice of zazen, the mind is stilled and the enslavement to the senses is broken—although temporarily.

Meditation aims at the elimination of the self, but it is not a descent into some incense-scented oblivion. Although all the cravings and selfish desires that make us dependent on the external world are eliminated in a process that has been described as the "ultimate loss of the self," which is the ultimate triumph of mind over matter, our consciousness remains unimpaired.

enlightenment

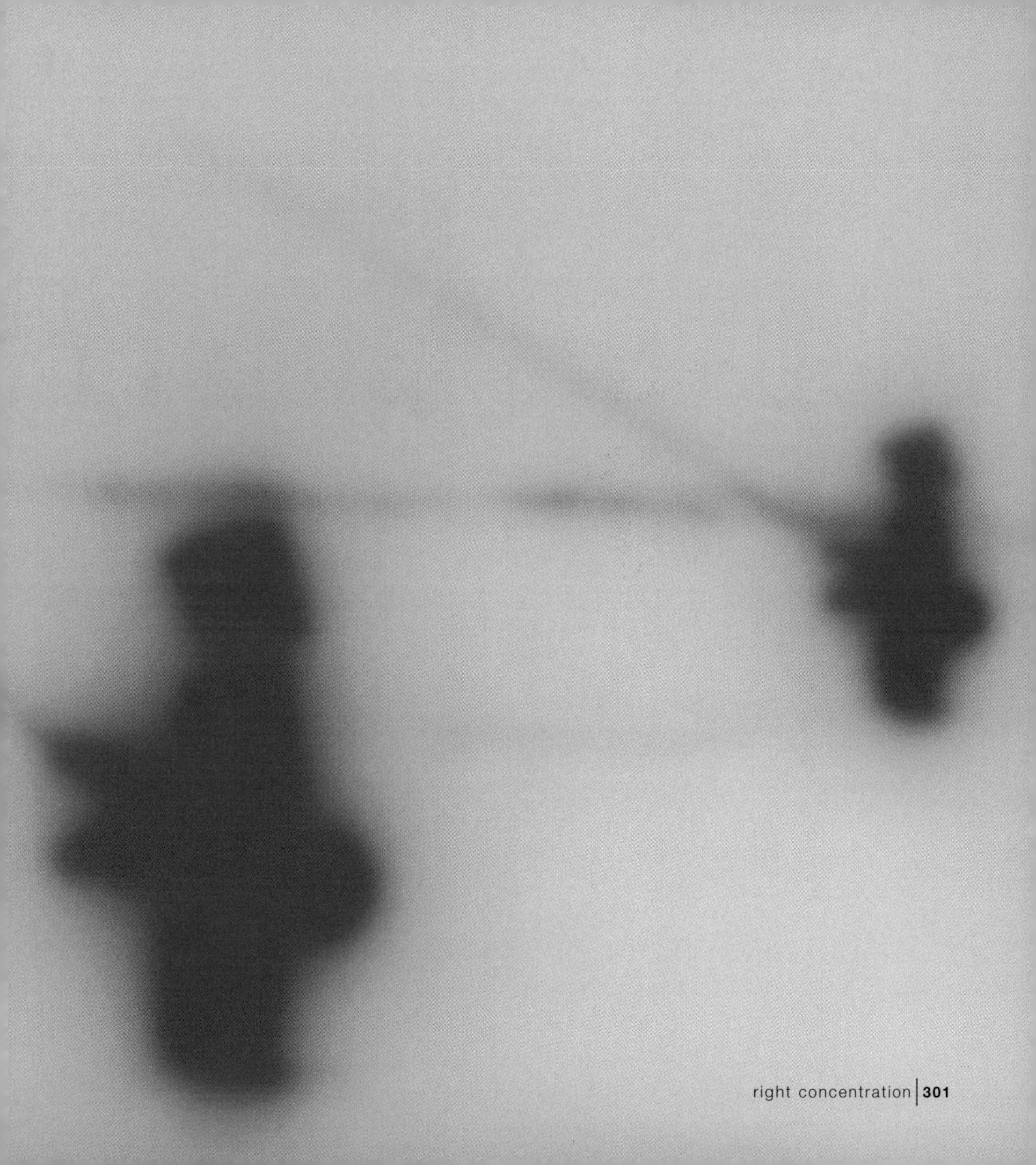

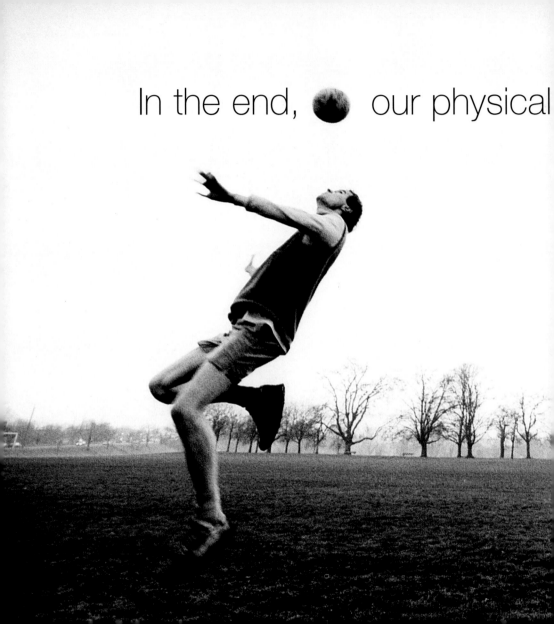

In the end, our physical

health, our painfully acquired
fitness will fail, but through
Zen, well-being will continue.

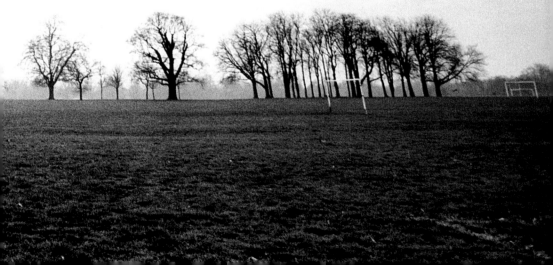

relaxation guidelines

Why meditation is effective is not well understood. According to Herbert Benson of the Harvard Medical School's Mind-Body Medical Institute, however, it is clear that it can elicit a "relaxation response" by which all the negative effects of stress on the body listed above are reduced or eliminated.

The problem with recommending exercise and relaxation techniques to combat stress is that there is no intuitive link between them. Although you can tell someone that their headaches, irritable bowel syndrome, or insomnia are caused by stress, making them "hear" it is another matter entirely. Listed on the following pages are some of the most common meditation techniques that can be used to control stress. It is impossible to give general guidelines for relaxation, but as an integral part of well-being, a relaxation exercise should form part of your daily routine.

preparations for meditation

clothing

Dress appropriately for the season. Remember, that when you're immobile, your body cools rapidly, even on a mild day. Wear layered clothing that you can remove easily in case of overheating. An overheated room will encourage drowsiness, so it is better to keep the temperature cool and dress accordingly.

location

This is only important in terms of what it must not be. For Zen meditation, you will need a plain environment, with no distracting colors or patterns around you.

time

Choose the quietest time of your day, which could be early morning before the household gets up, or mid-morning when everyone has gone out. You may meditate at any time, but avoid times when you are likely to be tired and drowsy, such as mid-afternoon and late evening.

food

It is advisable to meditate several hours before or after a large meal. Digestion takes a lot of energy and will encourage drowsiness. A light meal, however, is perfectly acceptable.

stimulants

Zen monks drink green tea to help them remain awake, but an excess of caffeine will make you jittery and may interrupt your practice. All other stimulants, such as alcohol and nicotine, will distort your experience of zazen.

posture

Most meditation techniques originated in cultures, such as Japan and India, where the chair was unknown or only used on ceremonial occasions or by the ruling elite. As a result, meditation is practiced sitting or kneeling on the ground (lying down is not considered a suitable position because it encourages drowsiness and sleep). This can prove a major stumbling block for many Westerners who are used to sitting in chairs and do not have the natural posture or leg flexibility to sit on the floor for more than a few minutes at a time.

In many traditions there is a belief that energy (chi in China, prana in India) travels through the body through channels and energy centers. It is important for the spine and head to be aligned so that the energy can flow smoothly. On a more practical level, it would be impossible to remain still in a seated position for an extended period if the body is twisted or slumped.

positions for meditation

full lotus

The king of positions, this locks the feet and legs together, and forms the most stable base for the body. However, it requires many years of stretching and practice before the position is comfortable.

Method: Bring the right foot on top of the left thigh, as close as possible to the body, and move the left foot onto the right thigh.

half lotus or cross-legged

Same as the full lotus, but the left foot is not lifted onto the right leg, but rests underneath it.

sei-za

This is the formal Japanese kneeling position. It requires good ankle flexibility to hold it for any length of time. A good way to practice sei-za is to kneel on one cushion with a smaller cushion (or cushions) under your buttocks to raise your body and relieve pressure on your ankles.

sitting

There is not reason why you should not practice meditation sitting on a chair. But it should be a straight-backed dining chair or a stool that will not allow you to slump. If you find it difficult to maintain a seated position with a straight back for any length of time, please consult an Alexander Technique teacher (see pages 106–127.)

breathing

Simple breathing exercises, such as abdominal breathing, have been shown to have a range of physical and mental benefits. Many of us pay little attention to our breathing, and especially under stress, we breathe shallowly and quickly, reducing the amount of oxygen available for the brain and body, and making us even less effective at dealing with the stressful situation. Use abdominal breathing as a preparation for meditation, to relax the body and center the mind.

abdominal breathing

1 In a quiet location and at a time when you will not be disturbed, sit with your head and body upright, your feet flat on the floor, and your hands resting easily on your thighs. Your body should be completely relaxed but alert, as if you could stand up at a moment's notice.

2 Dip your head forward slightly, close your eyes, and block out any other distractions around you. Breathing through your nose only, take a long deep breath, feeling the air slide over your palate and into your throat. Imagine that you are filling your lugs from the bottom up by relaxing your stomach muscles. Once the lower abdomen is full, fill your lungs by allowing your chest to expand out and up.

3 Once your lungs are completely full, hold the breath momentarily, before allowing it to escape. Empty your lungs from the top down—from the top of the lungs to the lower abdomen— allowing your chest to fall and then squeezing out the last of the air with your stomach muscles. Do not exaggerate the movement and strain to expel the last of the air. Keep the pressure smooth and constant. Try to breathe more deeply, slowly, and smoothly with each breath, until you can breathe in for a count of eight, and breathe out for a count of eight. Do not hold the breath in-between for more than a count of two until you have practiced the technique for some time. Stop if you feel any dizziness.

upper thoracic breathing

This technique is the opposite of abdominal breathing. Instead of releasing the abdomen to fill the lungs up with air, imagine that your navel and spine are tied with rope, and that you cannot expand the abdomen.

1 Pulling the abdomen in slightly as you breathe in, fill your lungs with air, and feel your breath lift your entire chest and back.

2 Hold for a moment, and release the breath, allowing your abdomen to relax slightly.

3 Continue in cycles of ten breaths.

meditation

external-focus meditation

This type of meditation, found across a range of religious cultures, including Christianity, uses an external stimulus, such as an image or sound, to focus the mind.

Buddhist and Hindu Tantric meditation techniques, one of which has been popularized in the West as Transcendental Meditation, uses the repetition of a mantra (symbolic incantation) and the contemplation of a mandala (diagrams) to remove the mind from the present to attain higher states of consciousness.

By engaging one of the major senses it is much easier to calm the mind, which will otherwise wander as boredom sets in. Although the original reason for these techniques was religious, they can be used to release stress.

exercise 1

1 Sit or kneel comfortably with your head and back erect, and your arms relaxed, hands resting on your thighs.

2 Breathe through your nose, slowly and easily. Close your eyes and repeat the syllable "Om" ("God" in Sanskrit) aloud. Extend the syllable on each repetition, trying to match it to your out breath.

3 Once your mind is calm and your breath relaxed, repeat the syllable silently in your mind. Continue for at least twenty minutes.

exercise 2

1 Sit or kneel as before with a mandala hanging in front of you at eye height. If you do not have a mandala, you may wish to use a devotional image connected to your own religious beliefs, or a complex, multicolored geometrical pattern.

2 Clearing your mind of all thoughts, observe the image until you think you will be able to remember it in detail. Then close your eyes and call the image back into your mind's eye. Try to hold the image for at least twenty minutes.

Internal-focus meditation

Several traditions use bodily processes such as breathing to
focus the mind. Toaism, which believes that life energy, chi,
circulates around the body, has developed a form of meditation
centered on the manipulation of chi.

exercise 3

1 Sit or kneel comfortably. Close your eyes. Imagine that there is
a circular channel in your body, going from your mouth, down
the front of your body, down to the base of the spine and up
your back to the crown of your head, and back to your mouth.
2 As you breathe in, imagine that you are absorbing chi with the
air, and direct it into the channel and around the body. Continue
breathing and circulating the chi for at least twenty minutes.

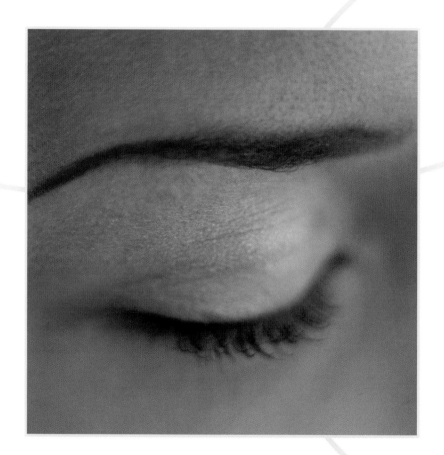

creative visualization

This is a modern, Western technique that has adapted ancient practices and put them to practical use, particularly in competitive sports. In creative visualization, an athlete can mentally "rehearse" an event or match, studying his technique, and anticipate a favorable outcome.

It can also used to control stress, but in this case the power of the imagination is used to transport the meditator to a world she has created for herself.

exercise 4

1 Sit or kneel comfortably. Close your eyes. Imagine you are at the gate of a garden. The garden is completely encircled by a high wall, and the gate is too high to see over. You can hear the trickling of water from streams, waterfalls, and fountains, hear the songs of birds, and feel the warm breeze that carries the scent of tropical flowers.

2 Push open the gates, and step into the garden. Stand and observe what you see before walking on. Continue your exploration of the garden for at least 20 minutes.

zazen

Often described as the most difficult form of meditation, zazen is deceptively simple in its practice. In a Zen meditation hall, the students are instructed to sit or kneel on cushions facing the wall. During a two-hour session, they will be expected to sit for between twenty and forty minutes before being given a ten-minute session of walking meditation. Zazen is difficult precisely because there is no external stimuli to hold the mind, which soon begins to wander.

exercise 5

1 Sit or kneel in a comfortable position facing a blank wall. There must be no object or image on the wall to distract your attention.

2 With your eyes open, begin to count your breaths until you reach ten and start over at one. If you lose count, or if your mind begins to wanders, begin the count at one. Continue for at least twenty minutes.

Designer: Simon Reece
Editor: Alison Moss

Sourcebooks, Inc.
P.O. Box 4410, Naperville, Illinois 60567-4410
(630) 961-3900
FAX: (630) 961-2168

Printed and bound in Italy by Amadeus
MQ 10 9 8 7 6 5 4 3 2 1

ISBN: 1-57071-687-0